SUICIDE BY SECURITY BLANKET, AND OTHER STORIES FROM THE CHILD PSYCHIATRY EMERGENCY SERVICE

Recent Titles in
The Praeger Series on Contemporary Health and Living

SUICIDE BY SECURITY BLANKET, AND OTHER STORIES FROM THE CHILD PSYCHIATRY EMERGENCY SERVICE

What Happens to Children with Acute Mental Illness

LAURA M. PRAGER, MD
AND ABIGAIL L. DONOVAN, MD

The Praeger Series on Contemporary Health and Living
Julie K. Silver, MD, Series Editor

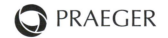 PRAEGER

AN IMPRINT OF ABC-CLIO, LLC
Santa Barbara, California • Denver, Colorado • Oxford, England

Library of Congress Cataloging-in-Publication Data

Prager, Laura M.
   Suicide by security blanket, and other stories from the child psychiatry
emergency service : what happens to children with acute mental
illness / Laura M. Prager and Abigail L. Donovan.
        p. ; cm. — (Praeger series on contemporary health and living)
   Includes index.
   ISBN 978-0-313-39949-7 (hardback : alk. paper) — ISBN 978-0-313-39950-3 (e-book)
   I. Donovan, Abigail L.   II. Title.   III. Series: Praeger series on contemporary health and living.
   [DNLM: 1. Massachusetts General Hospital.   2. Crisis Intervention—methods—
Massachusetts.   3. Emergency Services, Psychiatric—Massachusetts.   4. Child—
Massachusetts.   5. Mental Disorders—therapy—Massachusetts.   6. Self-Injurious
Behavior—Massachusetts. WS 350.2]
   LC Classification not assigned
   362.196'89009744—dc23   2012008767

ISBN: 978-0-313-39949-7
EISBN: 978-0-313-39950-3

16   15   14   13   12   1   2   3   4   5

This book is also available on the World Wide Web as an eBook.
Visit www.abc-clio.com for details.

Praeger
An Imprint of ABC-CLIO, LLC

ABC-CLIO, LLC
130 Cremona Drive, P.O. Box 1911
Santa Barbara, California 93116-1911

This book is printed on acid-free paper (∞)

Manufactured in the United States of America

To all of my family and friends—neither this book nor the work that I do every day would be possible without your encouragement. To my mother, Connie Donovan, and my brother, Brian Donovan—simple thanks do not seem adequate.

Liz Friedman and Jim Donovan deserve enormous gratitude for not only tirelessly reading each and every draft but also for being my biggest supporters. From the beginning, you believed in me. When I doubted myself, your belief only grew stronger.

Abigail L. Donovan

To Fred, Sam, and Lucia Millham—thank you for tolerating the innumerable calls from the APS with forbearance and humor and for making it possible for me to do more than I can do.

A special thanks to Susan Sacks Green who, since our freshman year in college, has been willing to read and edit anything I've written.

Finally, to my mother, Jane Price Prager, MD, who always answers the phone when I call.

Laura M. Prager

CONTENTS

Acknowledgments

Without the support of the incredible MGH/APS team of nurses, security guards, social workers, psychologists, attending physicians (psychiatrists, pediatricians, and emergency medicine doctors), and resource specialists, we cannot do our jobs and we could not have written this book. Thank you for being there all day, every day.

We are enormously grateful to our child patients and their families. To maintain complete privacy, all identifying details have been altered; many of the cases presented draw material from more than one patient's experience. We never record conversations between doctors and patients; each one is a reconstruction.

To the army of residents on the front line—thanks to each and every one of you for your willingness to learn along with us. We have often sent you back to obtain more of the patient's history (even when you think it's wasted effort), or asked you to make another phone call in search of collateral information, or demanded that you shift direction and follow a different path. Even though it is our job to teach you, the truth is that you have taught us just as much, if not more.

Heartfelt thanks go to our editor at ABC-CLIO, Debbie Carvalko, who took a chance on us and who has been supportive and encouraging at every step along the way.

INTRODUCTION

For the last decade, I have been the director of the Child Psychiatry Emergency Service at Massachusetts General Hospital (MGH). Until very recently, when Dr. Donovan joined the team, I ran the service by myself. I took calls almost every night, heard about almost every child who came through the doors of our Acute Psychiatry Service (APS), and shepherded both the adult resident on-site in the emergency room and the consulting child and adolescent psychiatry resident through the thought process that would lead them to a diagnosis, a treatment plan, and, ultimately, a disposition. These residents, who are in many different stages of training, learn to become both messenger and ambassador; they are on the front line, evaluating the patient, calling me to retell the story, then returning to the patient and offering the treatment plan we have concocted together. My family has become accustomed to my beeper going off at odd hours; over the years that plaintive alarm has receded into the background noise of our household and become no more than a slightly annoying yet familiar interruption.

Although I sometimes find the residents' presentations less than thorough, I never tire of hearing the stories. Psychiatric diagnosis and intervention depend primarily on the history or the story the patient tells. In the emergency room, one always starts with the question, "What makes today different from all other days?" That is, why did this child end up here today rather than yesterday, last week, or tomorrow? With that question and with all the other necessary questions that follow, no detail is insignificant. Trainees tease me about my interest in what they consider simply trivial matters, especially during what they think should be a rapid emergency room evaluation. What difference does it make if a family shows up during a school vacation week? Could it be that family members can only manage their bipolar child for a few days of constant togetherness before everyone runs out of energy and can no longer tolerate unpredictable hostility toward a younger sibling? Does it really matter if the 17-year-old boy who presents with new signs such as paranoia or auditory or visual hallucinations is a high school athlete? It matters a lot if he is a wrestler and decides to take diet pills to lose weight or, alternatively, to use anabolic steroids in a misguided attempt to increase muscle mass. One would hate to misdiagnose a delirium that stems from overuse of amphetamines (the active ingredient in medicines given for attention deficit disorder and also often found in diet pills) or "roid rage" as a new onset primary psychotic disorder. Who cares if the 10-year-old's mother has a driver's license and access to a car? We do, if we are considering hospitalizing the child in the only available inpatient bed that is located at least an hour and a half from his home.

And, just when I think I've heard everything, another child arrives at our door with an incomprehensible problem or, at the very least, a new take on an old problem. Nine-year-old children should not have marijuana metabolites in their urine toxicology screen; a 10-year-old boy should not have to consider strangling himself with his security blanket because his life is not worth living; 15-year-old girls should not have to switch from snorting heroin to injecting it in order to get someone's attention. Parents or other caretakers do not bring children to the emergency room simply because everyone involved has had a bad day. Something somewhere has gone very wrong. Imagine how desperate parents must be to show up, often in the middle of the night, admitting to us that they cannot manage their own child and fearing that we will not only agree with them but also take their child away. And, as I remind the residents at our weekly child rounds where the APS team reviews the child patients from the previous week, often enough, we do both.

Child psychiatry, whether practiced in the emergency room or in the relatively unhurried comfort of the clinic setting, is a field dependent on collateral information and bound by systems of care. The child is the identified patient but not always the only patient, and the emergency is usually in the eye of the beholder. The second grader sent directly to the APS because he is behaving like a chicken in the classroom and refusing to stop after many reminders to do so does not necessarily think that he has a psychiatric emergency, although the teacher may disagree. Children, for good or ill, come with parents or other custodial adults. They have teachers and guidance counselors, coaches and friends; they have pediatricians and sometimes therapists or psychopharmacologists. Those involved may have an important and informed perspective on the child's strengths and weaknesses. For the second-grade chicken, his clucking probably tells a crucial but limited part of the story. Our job is to figure out how to interpret his words, fill in the blanks with the impressions and observations of the adults who care for him, and then, like a high-stakes game of Mad Libs, create a narrative that explains the child's behavior and use that to guide our intervention.

What happens to the child, what services are available, and what level of care is accessible can sometimes depend more on the third party payer (insurance company) than on the clinical picture. Even if the child's difficulties could be managed by outpatient caregivers, they are so few and far between and so difficult to obtain that it is often easier to hospitalize a child on an inpatient psychiatric unit than to arrange for outpatient follow-up. Well-intentioned state initiatives created to provide community-based services for children such as in-home therapists, educational advocates, or after-school programs cannot meet the demand. Insurers offer such minimal remuneration for outpatient mental health services that hospitals and free-standing community clinics can offer such assistance only if they are willing to lose money or are underwritten by a hospital or a state agency. At the MGH, the entire Department of Child Psychiatry survives because the hospital administration is committed to supporting it. We are very lucky. Few institutions can or will do this. Fewer still will support a child psychiatry emergency service. As a result, children often come to the MGH APS from distant parts of Massachusetts or from other states. Designing a treatment plan for a child whose access to education, mental health, and ancillary services are governed by a totally different set of rules only magnifies the difficulties.

This book arises from my fascination with the endlessly complex stories of children's lives. It is so easy for a child living within some kind of psycho-social chaos to keep to himself, invisible and alone, until his problems, internal, external, or both, overwhelm his ability to cope. Most of these children cannot advocate for themselves, and many have no one else to advocate for them. My desire to tell their stories also arises out of my frustration with our current mental health system, one that consistently fails to meet the needs of children because to do so is too expensive and too time-consuming. It's a system in which insurers will pay for inpatient admissions but not for consistent outpatient services that might obviate the need for those admissions, a system where children must fail the least restrictive (read least expensive) level of care in order to qualify for a more intensive and much more expensive level of care, and a system in which children must come to an emergency room in crisis in order for someone to pay attention. This system reinforces the misguided belief that a child with mental health problems is not as acutely ill or as desperate for care as a child with other kinds of medical problems.

Over the years, I have seen hundreds of patients and heard about many, many more. Residents often ask me how I tolerate being paged day after day and night after night. The answer is that behind every call waits a child's story and a trainee's uncertainty. Both must be heard. Whether a child arrives in the emergency room strapped to a stretcher, carried by a parent, or on his or her own two feet, he or she should not leave without something changing—in his or her life, and in ours as well. We see these children in a moment of crisis, which offers us the opportunity to demand answers to previously unasked questions or shed a glaring light on a hidden vulnerability or tightly held secret. In the emergency setting, we wield enormous power: we can call for a state agency to investigate suspected parental abuse or neglect, physically restrain a child with leather straps, administer potent sedating medications, or commit a child to a locked unit against his or her will or the will of the parents. With that power comes responsibility; we must care for these children, keep them safe, and, despite the obstacles, help them and their families obtain the treatment they need. Sometimes we are successful; sometimes we are not. Here are their stories.

Laura M. Prager, MD
Boston, MA
Fall 2011

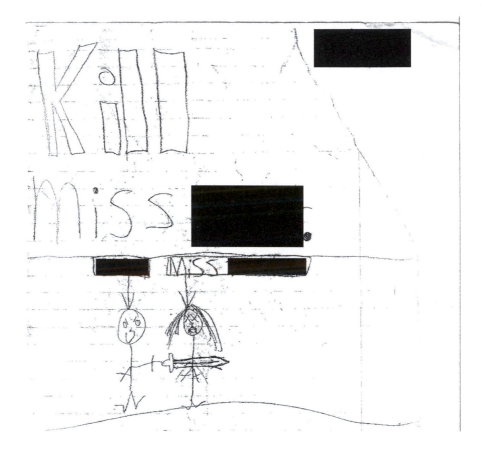

1

SAFE TO RETURN TO SCHOOL?

His name was Gabriel, but the chubby eight-year-old boy squirming slightly on a chair had not been billed as an angel. He had been sent directly from school to the Acute Psychiatry Service (APS) at the Massachusetts General Hospital (MGH) after he threatened to stab his second-grade teacher. The teacher, Miss Manchester, had discovered Gabriel drawing a picture that showed him happily impaling her with a knife. She was so upset that she snatched the drawing from Gabriel's desk, left the classroom, and ran to the vice principal's office brandishing the picture. The vice principal did not bother speaking with the little boy. He thought about calling 911 or the Boston Emergency Service Team's mental health crisis line, but instead he called Gabriel's mother to insist that she come right that minute to get her child and remove him from the premises. "We can't have our students threatening their teachers. I think Gabriel needs help," he said to the mother when she arrived. "You will need a doctor's note that says that he can safely return to school," were his parting words as she grabbed Gabriel by the hand and hustled him and his heavy backpack out the door and down the path to her car.

The MGH emergency room is a loud and bustling place—a maze of long, crowded hallways that connect different pods or sections. Each pod serves a different function, ranging from screening for those who feel sick but who may not really be sick to acute, for trauma patients or others who are critically ill. Pediatrics is decorated with vibrant, colorful murals of sea creatures on the floor and the walls; the waiting room there is referred to affectionately as the "guppy room." The Child Psychiatry Emergency Service does not have a pod of its own. All psychiatric patients, regardless of age, who do not appear to have active medical issues are diverted through another door into a private area with another waiting room and an adjacent locked area. The locked unit consists of four interview rooms, three holding rooms in which volatile patients can be safely interviewed and observed, and a larger open area with a couch and a television set. Within the unit, nurses, psychiatry residents, and security guards work side by side. Four residents in their second year of training, junior residents, rotate through the unit every three months; a senior resident, one in his or her third or fourth year of training, comes into work overnight, side by side with the junior who has been designated as the night float; an attending who is an adult psychiatrist is also present and runs the show from 8 A.M. until 10 P.M. A nurse-practitioner, psychology intern, or medical student may also be working there at any given time. After evaluating a child patient (one who is under the age of 18), the adult resident, nurse-practitioner, psychology intern, or med student will then call a child psychiatry resident (someone in his or her fifth or sixth year out of medical school) to discuss the case. The MGH is one of the only hospitals in the country in which a patient of any age can be evaluated at any hour of the day or night by a psychiatric resident, an attending psychiatrist, and, if young enough, by a child psychiatry resident and/or an attending child psychiatrist.

Although rules established by the state mandate the separation of children under the age of 18 from adults within the locked evaluation unit, no such rules apply to the waiting room; there, young children mingle freely with, among others, penniless drug addicts looking for something to stem their craving, homeless people looking for a warm place to sit and a ride to a shelter, or newly released prisoners seeking mental health services. It was in that room on one of the stained green chairs pushed up in a row against the wall that Gabriel sat with his mother, waiting for the psychiatrist who he hoped would listen to his story and then write the note saying that he could safely return to school.

The wait would be at least several hours. Gabriel and his mother sat quietly as patients filed in and out. Occasionally, the locked door would click open and a doctor or nurse would call someone's name; that person would get up and follow. Sometimes, the patients came back out—sometimes they didn't. No one seemed particularly concerned that Gabriel had been accused of threatening to kill his teacher. The nurse, a friendly woman with blond hair cascading over her shoulders, interviewed him briefly when he first checked in and simply asked his mother if she felt they could manage waiting in the waiting room. When his mother looked at him with her eyebrows raised, he nodded yes. Then the nurse quickly took his pulse and blood pressure and ran a fancy thermometer over his forehead that she told him measured his temperature. She wrote all the results down on a piece of paper.

"You won't run away now, will you?" she said with a wink. "Let me know if you need something to eat."

That was that. The wait began.

Gabriel got bored after a while with nothing to do but swing his legs and stare at the other people sitting there. Some of them were crying; some stared blankly off into space. No one met his eye. One woman sat calmly knitting something purple. She had bags full of what looked like clothes tucked under her chair. The man in the corner kept falling asleep and then slipping out of his chair; he would swear and then pick himself up and sit back down. Occasionally, he left the waiting room for a few minutes at a time and then returned smelling of cigarette smoke.

Soon Gabriel told his mother he was hungry. After she told the receptionist, a pleasant young woman wearing a pink coat and a pin announcing her
volunteer status brought each of them a turkey sandwich and a juice box in a
brown paper bag. There was still nothing to do. His mother sat with her eyes
closed, head in her hand. Finally, Gabriel remembered that he had his pencils
and papers in his backpack. He opened it up and started to pull things out. He
was worried. He never should have been drawing instead of listening to what
Miss Manchester was telling the class. But she wasn't his real teacher; she was
only filling in for his real teacher who had left to have a baby. Miss Manchester
just didn't know how tough it was for him to read the books everyone else was
reading. He had tried to tell her that he was supposed to be reading a different
book, but she was too busy to listen.

The resident, Dr. G, arrived for a four-hour shift. A pediatrician in his second year of training, he was in the midst of a rotation designed to teach him
about psychiatric problems in children. One afternoon a week he joined the
junior psychiatry residents in the APS, hoping that there would be a patient
under 18 needing evaluation so that he could gain some experience. Among
the long list of patients on the dry-erase board in the back room where the
doctors sat busily entering information into computers, Dr. G read that Gabriel
was eight years old, that he was apparently planning to kill his second-grade
teacher, and that his mother wanted a note for school. He checked in with the
attending psychiatrist and wrote his initials beside Gabriel's name on the board
so the other residents would know that he was taking the case.

Eight-year-olds are fun to interview, as most love to talk about themselves.
They are generally eager to please, engaged in mastering new skills and com-
paring themselves to their friends, quick to insist that everyone has to follow
the same rules, and quick to complain if the rules are not fair. The problem is
that, despite their willingness to talk freely, eight-year-olds tell stories that may
have nothing to do with why they are in the emergency room. Their perspective
on what has landed them in this predicament is rarely the same as that of the
adults who are worried about them. A child who says he wanted to die when
he was the last one picked for floor hockey can help us understand that he feels
badly about his athletic prowess and/or that he is not well-liked by his peers.
Yet, we could not expect that same child to describe his long-standing delays
in fine and gross motor development, coordination, and age-appropriate social
interactions—information that helps to place his experience in gym in a different
framework. The child's view is important—but it is only one piece of the puzzle.

For these reasons, sometimes it is more helpful to hear from a parent or
other caregiver before talking one-on-one with the child. But, in this case, there
was no way that Dr. G could leave Gabriel alone in what seemed to be a more
than unsavory waiting room. He grabbed the "Child Template," which listed all
the questions he was supposed to ask during an interview of this type, flashed
his ID badge at the security lock inside the unit, opened the door to the waiting room, and called the child's name. Gabriel and his mother followed him
through the locked door and into an interview room.

Interview rooms are quite small and uncomfortable with uniformly dirty beige walls and floor, usually furnished with two or three blue chairs and a desk bolted to the wall. There are no frills, no soft edges, and no colorful pictures, only the bright, unforgiving glare of fluorescent ceiling lights. Gabriel took one chair, his mother another, and the doctor the third. Then Dr. G started at the beginning: name, age, address, insurance company, legal guardian. All of that information was, of course, already stored somewhere in the hospital database, but asking the questions directly sometimes has added benefits. An emergency room evaluation, for better or worse, has one goal: disposition. In order to guide the patient to the next stop, you have to know where he started. Like those board games, aptly named Sorry or Trouble, which kids in Gabriel's age group love to play—if you land on the wrong square, you have to go all the way back to the beginning. With child psychiatry in particular, geography can shape destiny. It's not helpful to admit a child to a hospital or refer him to a clinic that is located far from his home. Family members may not even be able to get there, let alone participate actively in treatment. If the patient is lucky enough to live in a town with a high tax base, there will likely be more services available, either within the school setting or from other community-supported resources. If he isn't, resources may be impossible to come by. Knowing where the patient comes from lets the interviewer consider options for disposition at the same time as he is learning about the problem.

"My name is Gabriel," answered Gabriel. "I live in Revere."

"No, you don't," interjected his mother, "You live in Winthrop. We just moved," she explained apologetically. "He forgets."

Gabriel blinked.

"Did you have to switch schools when you moved, Gabriel?" Dr. G asked him.

"No," mother answered again. "I asked special permission for him to continue at the same school that he's been attending since he was in kindergarten, at least until the end of the school year. I have to drive him, but it's not far. I just don't understand what happened today. He has been doing so well. He used to have tantrums at school all the time, but he has been much, much better. He even has a good friend in his class this year. I don't think he's done anything bad, not really. The vice principal says that he threatened Miss Manchester, but I don't believe it. He's not that kind of boy. He wouldn't hurt anyone. He loves to draw," she added as an afterthought, "I think it was his drawings that caused the problem."

"Can you tell us what happened today?" Dr. G asked Gabriel.

"I drew a bad picture," he muttered, looking down at his legs, which didn't quite reach the floor.

"What was bad about it?"

"I was mad at Miss Manchester. It wasn't nice."

"Can you show it to me?"

Gabriel started rustling around in his backpack.

"Why were you so mad at her?"

"It was reading. We were having reading. I'm supposed to be reading about Clifford, but she gave me a chapter book."

"*Clifford the Big Red Dog?*" The resident had suddenly remembered the cartoon in which a large red dog parades around a town doing good deeds.

For the first time, Gabriel looked up. He smiled shyly at Dr. G. "Yeah. Clifford. I like Clifford. She told me I was too old for Clifford and I should read something else."

"Gabriel has a learning disability," his mother said. "Reading is difficult for him. He gets special help. His regular teacher, Mrs. S, works with him on reading. I don't know why Miss Manchester didn't remember that."

"But I thought Miss Manchester was the teacher?" Dr. G asked.

"She's the assistant teacher. She's very young, but she's filling in because Mrs. S is out having a baby."

Gabriel suddenly hopped out of his chair and began to move somewhat aimlessly around the room. "I was mad," he said, and his eyes filled with tears. "I drew a picture. I was really mad, and so I thought about stabbing Miss Manchester with a knife." He went back to his chair, reached into his backpack, and pulled out a sheaf of papers.

"Here," he said, thrusting a piece of paper into Dr. G's hand.

"I drew this and Miss Manchester got really upset. She almost started to cry. I didn't want her to cry. I was just mad." Tears ran down the boy's cheeks. He ran to his mother and hid his face on her shoulder. She put her arm around him.

"He's not a bad boy," she said. "He's never hurt anyone. He never even gets into fights with the other kids. They sometimes make fun of him, but he never does anything."

Dr. G looked at Gabriel's mother and then at Gabriel.

"What does your picture mean?" Dr. G asked him.

"I was so mad that I wanted to hurt her. See, I took a big knife and I hurt her with it. See, she is crying."

"So after Miss Manchester got upset, then what happened?"

"I drew another picture," he mumbled into his mother's shoulder.

"You drew another picture? Can I see that one, too?"

"I didn't really want to hurt Miss Manchester. I was just mad at her." Gabriel sat down on the floor. "It was just a picture," he said after a bit.

"Where is the other picture?"

Gabriel pulled his backpack toward him and started taking everything out. Soon, amidst his crumpled papers, he found another sheet that he handed to his mother.

"She was crying, so I drew this," he said.

"Did Miss Manchester see this second picture?" asked Dr. G.

"No," replied Gabriel. "She ran out of the room before I could show it to her." He leaned forward and put his head in his hands.

"You see," said mother, "I told you that Gabriel was a good kid."

"I like Miss Manchester," he said, lifting his head up to look at Dr. G. Then he added, shyly, "I thought she liked me, too. I knew I had made her upset.

I wanted to make up. That's what you do," he asked Dr. G, "isn't it? It was just a picture. I didn't really hurt her. She's my teacher. I don't want to hurt her. Sometimes she's nice."

* * *

Scary drawings are the catalyst for many children's emergency room visits. This is the post-Columbine, post–Virginia Tech era, marked by several highly publicized and devastating school shootings and, in Massachusetts, the fairly recent stabbing death of one high school student at the hands of another. Teachers and administrators are understandably afraid to interpret violent drawings and reach conclusions about their students' ideas or fantasies, capabilities or intentions. While it is usually teenagers who draw graphic images of dismemberment or mass destruction, on occasion elementary school children are referred for similar reasons. There is little if any evidence that children's violent drawings portend violent action, but that fact can be difficult to remember when one is faced with these dramatic and sometimes gory pictures. School administrators and even seasoned therapists often demand an emergency psychiatric evaluation when confronted with their students' or patients' explicit or powerful drawings.

Not all children sent directly to the ED from school with the question "safe to return?" stamped on their registration packet come with the answer to that question sketched on notebook paper in black and white. Drawings are usually only an admission ticket; they must be understood in the context of the child's developmental stage and social environment. After Dr. G met with Gabriel and his mother, he spoke with the attending psychiatrist and then called the vice principal to talk about what had happened and discuss how he might help teacher and student to mend their fences. Luckily, Gabriel was just an eight-year-old with a learning disability, perhaps somewhat less mature than many of his second-grade classmates, who was embarrassed that he read less well than other members of his class. When his teacher shamed him, he got upset and angry and drew a picture to express his feelings. But Gabriel had strengths; he had the ability to manage those feelings by drawing pictures, not by throwing a tantrum, or running out of the classroom, or hurting himself or anyone else. He knew his picture would hurt his teacher's feelings. To make amends, he quickly drew another one to show that, even though he was mad, he still loved her. He had experienced intense and disturbing emotions: he wanted both to hurt her as he had been hurt and to love her the way he wanted to be loved. In an effort to master his feelings and prevent himself from acting in a way that he knew was reprehensible, Gabriel drew a picture of his fantasies, both the good and the bad. Not only did he draw them clearly, he was willing to talk about them when asked.

If only all school-age children sent to the emergency room directly from school could tell a story like Gabriel's, one in which child development played out in all its glory right in front of our eyes. The question of whether or not Gabriel was safe to return to school was easy to answer. For many children, it is not. Gabriel's drawings were not the problem, they were the solution. His mother and, later, his other teachers described Gabriel as a sweet boy who was liked by his classmates; he used to have tantrums when frustrated and upset in which he cried and occasionally sucked his thumb, but he had matured over the past year and rarely got upset in class despite his ongoing struggles with reading. He had never hurt anyone before, nor had anyone hurt him; the likelihood that he would do something dangerous in his second-grade classroom was low.

School administrators and teachers often demand that a child psychiatrist write a note documenting that a child who has voiced threatening statements or written or drawn scary stories or pictures can remain safe at school. But an emergency room evaluation captures only a discrete moment in time, a cross section rather than longitudinal view. No psychiatrist, regardless of experience or skill, can, after one interview, predict a patient's future actions, not even those of an eight-year-old with a penchant for drawing. No child leaves the APS with a note guaranteeing that he can be safely at school; there are no guarantees. In Gabriel's case, Dr. G recommended that the teacher and the vice principal meet with Gabriel, listen to his entire story, and then make a judgment as to whether or not they could welcome him back to the class. The decision as to whether or not Gabriel was safe in the second grade ultimately rested with the school. Would Miss Manchester, the object of his anger and admiration, continue to worry that Gabriel would come after her or would she be able to understand the conflicted, intense feelings of her student and appreciate them as an example of a normal developmental stage? Would she be willing to try to work with him, perhaps in conjunction with a school social worker or psychologist, in order to help Gabriel express his feelings differently? Let's hope so. Gabriel was certainly no angel, but he wasn't a demon, either.

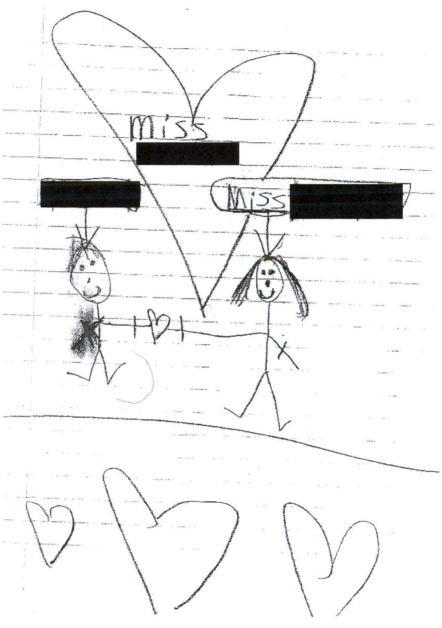

2

GHOSTLY DRAWINGS

Most five-year-olds like to draw, and sometimes they like to draw on themselves. No one thought much of it when Helena arrived at her kindergarten class on a Tuesday morning in the spring with dark squiggles in ballpoint pen covering her forearms and her feet and ankles. She had also used magic markers to create a pretend toenail polish. The teacher sent her to the nurse's office, and the nurse helped her to scrub her arms and legs clean. When asked about the markings, Helena first told the teacher that a ghost named Cynthia had drawn them, and then she said that really it was her mom who had drawn them, and finally she said that she had drawn them herself.

The next day, Helena's arms and legs had only faint residual markings. The school nurse checked in on her mid-morning, and Helena skipped happily up to her. Without hesitating a bit, Helena pulled down her pants to show the nurse some new dark, complex intersecting lines, both curves and straight edges, with triangular areas fully colored in, extending from her upper, inner thighs, just below her underwear, all the way down to her knees. Again, the little girl wasn't exactly clear about who had done the drawings; maybe a ghost, maybe mom, or maybe she had done the deed herself when she could not sleep at night.

The nurse didn't feel as happy about the drawings as Helena. In fact, she was not at all happy. Little girls should not have ballpoint pen all over their inner thighs. She asked the child to wait in the office while she called her mother to tell her about the new drawings and to suggest that she take Helena to see her pediatrician. The nurse thought that those drawings were just a little bit too intricate to have been drawn by a kindergarten artist, not to mention that they covered parts of her body that should be private.

Mother called the pediatrician, explained the urgency of her call, and asked for a same-day appointment. She was able to schedule a mid-afternoon time with one of the doctors in the practice. Once there, mother acknowledged that she had glimpsed the drawings early that morning, but did not appreciate how extensive and elaborate they were, and had assumed that Helena had again drawn on herself. She sent her to school without further investigation. She had never observed Helena actually using a ballpoint pen on her skin, but she couldn't think of an alternative explanation. It was only the two of them at home, and she vehemently denied that she herself had ever drawn on her child.

The covering doctor was puzzled, too. She didn't know Helena well. According to the medical record, Helena's most recent visit was in November of the previous year, when mother had brought her in for an annual physical exam. At that time, the pediatrician had noted that she was active, bright, engaging, and growing normally. The covering doctor admitted that she couldn't offer much, but she agreed with the school nurse that the drawings looked too complex for a five-year-old to have drawn on herself. When she asked the same question everyone else had asked, Helena told her that "ghosts did it." Then the doctor suggested that the mother take Helena for an emergency psychiatric evaluation, called the ED, and sent the two on their way.

Helena and her mother showed up a bit after 5 P.M. Almost change of shift. Helena was wearing a pink shirt with flowers on it, purple pants with an elastic waist, and open sandals. Her orange-colored toenails peeped through the openings in the sandals; her hair was pulled back in a ponytail. She hopped and skipped her way through the locked door from the waiting room to the large room in the back of the secured area of the APS that contained a couch, a few chairs, and a TV. Mother was wearing a suit. She kept pulling the skirt down as she walked behind Helena, her high heels clicking on the tile floor.

Mother and Helena settled down to wait. Mother politely inquired if there was some way that she could get Helena something to eat as it was almost dinner time. The nurse told mother that she was expecting the dinner trays to come up within the next 30 minutes and that the entree was likely to be macaroni and cheese. Both Helena and mother appeared quite happy about that.

"When will the doctor see us?" mother asked.

"Soon, I hope," was the answer.

Helena found the markers and stack of plain printer paper that one of the nursing assistants had brought and placed on the table between the two chairs and announced to no one in particular that she was going to write a chapter book about the park near her home. Mother explained to the assistant that Helena loved going to the park and that she kept asking when it would be summer time again.

It was only an hour later when both the junior and senior residents on call that evening sat down to talk with Helena and her mother. Helena's aunt arrived at about the same time, bringing Helena a stuffed rabbit that Helena took from her eagerly and cradled in her arms, cooing "Bunny" to herself very softly as she pranced around the room.

The two doctors decided to divide and conquer. One stayed to talk with Helena, and the other brought mother to an interview room to talk.

"See if you can get Helena to draw," the senior told the junior. "When I spoke with the attending, she asked if Helena were even capable of drawing the complex design that's on her body."

Helena grabbed her mother's arm and started to cry as mother started to follow the resident down the hall. The aunt came between them and told Helena, "There, there. Mommy is just going to talk with the doctor and then she'll be right back."

To the doctor, she said, "Helena hates it when her mother isn't with her. Ever since her mother was sick last year, she's been like this."

"Mommy is fine, now," she said to Helena, and the little girl allowed herself to be soothed, hugged Bunny again, and went back to the little table where she had been drawing.

"What happened to Helena's mother?" the resident asked the aunt.

"She was in a car accident last year and had to be in the hospital for a few nights. It was very traumatizing for Helena."

The junior resident sat down on one of the chairs beside Helena. "What are you drawing?" he asked.

"Book," she said. She held up the picture proudly. On one side of a piece of white printer paper she had written "HELENA WEN TO THE PAK" in block letters.

"Did you go to the park?" the resident asked her.

"I went to the park," she said and she resumed drawing.

"Helena loves to go to the park," the aunt chimed in. "She has a pail and a shovel for the sandbox and she's a very good little climber. She is also good at writing and drawing," she added as an afterthought.

Helena nodded vigorously as she drew. "Want to see my other drawings?" she demanded suddenly.

Without prompting, she pulled down her pants and turned her knees slightly in order to display her upper thighs, which were covered with ballpoint pen lines and squiggles with intersecting lines creating spaces that were carefully filled in. The lines were dark, the curves were smooth, and the pen markings in the spaces were confluent.

The resident had already heard that Helena gave several different answers to the question about who had drawn on her legs. It didn't seem like it was worth it to ask the same question again.

Helena saved him the trouble.

"My mommy told me to do it," she announced.

"Do what?"

"The drawings," she said, and patted her stomach.

"Why did she tell you to do that?"

"She just said to."

"What did you draw?"

"Scary penguin," she said.

"Scary penguin? Who is that?"

"Scary penguin."

"Is this scary penguin?" the resident picked up Helena's pink stuffed bunny. "No. Of course not," she said. "That's Bunny."

Helena took a new sheet of paper, drew a medium-sized circle, and started to put a very small stick figure inside of it. "I went to the park," she said again.

"Is that the park?" the resident asked as he pointed to the large circle.

"Yup. My mommy and I went together. Here is mommy," and she drew another tiny stick figure. Then she made some small squares that she explained were swings.

"Sounds like you and your mommy have fun together," said the resident.

The aunt chimed in, "They do have fun, especially now that it's just the two of them. Helena's father hasn't been around much."

* * *

Down the hall, the senior resident sat with Helena's mother. Soon the child psychiatry resident joined him. The unwritten rule was that the child psychiatry residents who serve as consultants to the ED must actually interview every child under the age of 10, not just offer recommendations for management over the phone as they might do with a pre-teen or adolescent. The MGH is a teaching hospital. Child psychiatry residents also need practice with hands-on emergency assessments of very young children and their families.

The two residents stepped out of the interview room and the senior resident filled the child psychiatry resident in on what he knew. "I don't know what the big fuss is about," he said. "The kid is five; she drew on her legs. This needs an ED visit?"

The child psychiatry resident pointed out the problem was that the child had given several different explanations as to who did the drawings. And, no one was sure that Helena could have done the drawings herself given their location and complexity. All in all, it was a mystery.

"You think this is abuse?" he asked.

"I don't know what to think," she said. "I've never seen anything like this before, and neither has my attending; I asked her. Unless we can get a really good explanation, we'll probably have to file with the Department of Children and Families (DCF). It's just too weird."

* * *

DCF is the state agency charged with protecting the health and well-being of all the children in the Commonwealth of Massachusetts. If a caregiver (doctor, nurse, teacher, police officer, day care worker, social worker, etc.) suspects that a child is being abused or neglected, he or she is required by law to inform DCF. Abuse includes either physical injury or serious emotional injury. Reporting a suspicion to the agency is called filing a 51A, because the law is found in Section 51A of the Massachusetts General Law Chapter 119. There is a fine for failure to file; there is no fine for filing. Once the paperwork has been filed, DCF must review or screen the case within 24 hours and decide whether to investigate the allegation further.

APS residents file many 51A's. Sometimes the situation is dire and the child in acute danger. In such cases, the course is clear. But, defining what constitutes abuse or neglect can be difficult and confusing. That task belongs to DCF. The psychiatry resident's job is to alert the state agency if he or she suspects that a child is experiencing physical or emotional injury, or if the child's basic needs have been neglected, and then do everything he or she can to keep the child safe.

* * *

Helena's mother started crying almost as soon as she sat down in one of the chairs in the interview room. She was angry with herself for having sent Helena to school with the pen drawings; she was sure that Helena had drawn them.

"When I asked her before school, Helena told me that a ghost named Cynthia had drawn on her with a pen. I knew that she was lying, but she's been doing a lot of lying lately. A couple of nights ago, she stayed up after I tucked her in, drew on her arms with a pen she found in my purse, and then came down to show me. She told me a ghost had done it. I thought it was funny at first." She stopped talking and wiped the tears from her eyes. A few minutes went by in silence.

"This all has to do with her father," she said.

Helena's parents had separated shortly after Helena was born, as father was both verbally and emotionally abusive toward mother. Father rarely visited Helena during the first few years of her life; in fact, mother thought perhaps he had moved away, and she was relieved. Since then, she had worked full time to support herself and Helena, asking nothing from Helena's father. However, within the last six months, he had reappeared in the area and gone to court to demand visitation rights. The court awarded him supervised visits, and Helena had had six visits with him under supervision by a social worker within the last few months. The most recent visit with father had been four days earlier. Father was not happy that the visits were supervised and told the mother that he was planning to challenge that ruling and demand unsupervised visits.

Since resuming visits with father, Helena had appeared more moody (occasionally crying at home for no apparent reason) and had had increased difficulty separating from her mother. She had long slept in her mother's bed at night with mother and Bunny for company. The usual routine involved climbing into bed and having mother read a story before she went back downstairs. However, within the last few months, Helena had had more difficulty falling asleep unless her mother stayed with her. After several years of being dry at night, she had also begun to wet the bed. Mother attributed these changes to father's reappearance in her child's life, and she had gone to court a few days earlier, while Helena was in school, to ask the judge that his visits be terminated.

"He's nothing but trouble," she added.

"Who?" asked the child psychiatry resident.

"Helena's father."

"Why do you say that?" the resident asked.

"He just is," the mother answered but didn't elaborate further. Mother had regained her composure. "I assure you that I didn't draw on my own child," she continued. "I think Helena must have done it herself. She's a smart little girl and she certainly loves to draw. I can't think of anything else."

"What happened after you went to court?"

"They continued the case. Judge wasn't listening to me. Helena's father still has supervised visits for the next few months and then we go back."

* * *

Around the corner, Helena continued to draw and talk with the junior resident and her aunt. She informed them that her picture book would have four pages. She decided to make another page, which she entitled Chapter 1. She then drew a picture of a girl with long curly hair and smiling face.

The resident complimented her on her drawings. "Is that girl supposed to be you?" he asked.

"She has long curly hair. I have straight hair," Helena pointed out.

"I don't suppose that you could draw a picture for me just like the squiggles that you or the ghost or your mother drew on your legs?" he asked.

Helena didn't answer but took another sheet of printer paper and started drawing furiously. She dashed straight lines across the page and then made another set so that the lines crossed each other at angles, muttering, "Good. Yup," as she drew. She did not fill in the shapes made by the intersecting lines, nor were the lines she drew rounded or smooth.

"Is this the same as what is on your legs?"

She bent down to add to the orange color on her toenails, and her face was hidden.

"Helena," the resident continued, "does this drawing look like what is on your legs?"

"I don't know," she said.

He tried one more time, "Who did the drawings on your legs?"

Helena looked directly at him, "A ghost named Cynthia, " she said.

"Not you? I thought you said your mother told you to do them?"

"That was before."

"Before?"

Helena shook her head vigorously back and forth as if to say no, no, no. "I did some before. Cynthia did some, too."

"But before what?"

"Before I came here," Helena sighed with exasperation. "Can I go home now?"

* * *

Stalemate. Who drew on Helena? Mother? Helena? Cynthia, the ghost? Father?

Mother blamed Helena; Helena blamed herself, her mother, and a ghost. Where does the truth lie? And, as the senior resident asked, does it really matter?

Yes, it matters. Drawing all over the inner thighs of a young girl is complicated business. None of the adults who heard the story felt comfortable. Each had the suspicion that these drawings represented some kind of inappropriate closeness between this five-year-old girl and an adult, which is why the child and her mother were sent from the school to the pediatrician's office to the ED. Everyone was worried, but no one wanted to make a false accusation or, worse, miss a latent danger.

If, in fact, Helena drew on herself, how did she do it and why? Was it, as mother suggested, due to the reappearance of her father and his ongoing visits? The drawings, coupled with her increasing difficulty with separation from her mother as manifested by difficulty falling asleep by herself at bedtime and the new onset of wetting the bed at night, suggest a high degree of confusion and stress. Both types of behavior represent regression. Helena seemed to have forgotten the developmentally appropriate tasks she had already mastered—her ability to put herself to sleep and to stay dry at night—and begun to demonstrate behaviors more characteristic of younger children. But why?

Mother's allegation that her ex-husband was nothing but trouble added another wrinkle. Yet, mother had presented only her side of the story. It was not clear whether father was "trouble," and even if he were, whether that would affect his relationship with his young daughter. His visits were supervised; what could have been happening within that time frame that might have caused Helena to cover herself with pen lines? We do not know what father said to her during the visits, but, again, as someone else was listening, how bad could it have been?

Helena also said that mother had either (1) told her to draw on herself or (2) done the drawings. Why would mother want to draw on Helena? Could it have been part of a game that the two were playing, and now mother was too embarrassed to admit that? Could mother have wanted to create this mystery in order to cast blame on the father and gain points with the judge as part of her attempt to terminate the father's rights? Did mother tell Helena to draw on herself and then help her to color the spaces in between the lines in order to make the drawings more dramatic? Mother may have been lying about her role in the drawings, but she did share that she and Helena's father were at odds and admit that her current agenda was to terminate his visits because she felt he was upsetting Helena.

Furthermore, could Helena have actually drawn on herself? In other words, was it physically possible? Did she have the requisite fine motor skills to do so? The answer to those questions, too, was not clear. She may have been able to create complicated line drawings, but she did not demonstrate that ability in the ED. Her chapter book was age appropriate—a simple figure drawing with a smiling face giving the impression that she, too, was a happy girl. Another drawing in which the stick figures and swings were the same size and seemingly floating in space was an age-appropriate depiction. Could she actually have duplicated the elaborate, smooth scribbles present on her legs if she had wanted to, or did that demand fine motor skills that she didn't yet possess?

And why was it so difficult to get a straight story from Helena? Helena wasn't exactly lying; she was telling her version of the truth. Sometimes when kids this age lie, it is in the service of protecting themselves. So it's possible that Helena chose to blame someone else, that is, her mother or a ghost, for the drawings in order to shift the responsibility and avoid punishment.

The resident did not challenge her story about the ghost. He might have asked what she thought about ghosts in order to figure out if she really still believed in ghosts or whether some part of her knew that they were just pretend. Sometimes kids Helena's age use fantasy as a way of handling intense emotions. Was Cynthia the ghostly representation of fright, the embodiment of her fear of what had happened to her, whether driven by her own need to draw on herself or by someone else's need to do it?

And, after all of this conjecture, what do we recommend? Can she go home now?

The decision: yes—she can go home. We have some suspicions that the relationship among mother, father, and Helena is changing, some worries that Helena is either being used as a bargaining chip or that someone is actually touching her in ways she considers invasive and frightening. When Helena pulled down her pants to show us her drawings, perhaps she was encouraging us to look under the brightly colored clothing and glimpse the darker, amorphous, ghostly design that lay beneath.

* * *

The APS residents filed a 51A with DCF and referred Helena and her mother to the MGH Outpatient Clinic for an urgent evaluation. The DCF worker opened the case, but could not determine the identity of the artist and closed the case within weeks.

* * *

In this case, as with many APS cases, we did the best we could at the time: asked questions, raised concerns, involved DCF, and tried to ensure close follow-up on the outpatient basis. Rarely, if ever, do we learn what happens when the patient leaves the ED and heads for her next stop, whether it is to the confines of an inpatient psychiatric unit or, as in this case, to her home. The image of the intricate pen drawings remains as a tangible, horrifying reminder of how difficult it is to identify or prove abuse—our conclusion as ambiguous as the squiggles and swirls that covered Helena's legs.

3

A Wounded Son

Bhanu and his father arrived at the ED several hours ago, after Mr. Patel received a phone call from Bhanu's school. They told him that his son had to see a psychiatrist right away, or they would take him to court. He wasn't really sure they could do that, but he also wasn't really sure they couldn't, so he brought Bhanu in to the MGH emergency department and asked for the psychiatrist. He was told they would have to wait several hours, but what else could he do? He didn't want Bhanu to get in trouble with the law.

So, they sat in the crowded waiting room, side by side. Bhanu, dressed in a faded green sweat suit, kept his head down, staring at the floor. His dark hair was dirty and fell limply across his forehead. His thin frame was downright bony now, and sharp elbows and knees poked through the pilled fabric of his sweat suit. His father sat straight in the chair beside him, a small, thin man himself. He kept his head up and his eyes forward—alert for the sound of their names being called.

Bhanu had always been the odd kid out. He had spent the first eight years of his life in India and then moved to Boston because his parents wanted a better life for themselves and for him. The transition to America was hard for both of his parents, but especially for his mother, who had to work nights cleaning an office building, and so she spent most of her days asleep. Bhanu learned English by watching cartoons, and now, even at the age of 13, he still used phrases like "ya-ba-da-ba-doo!" from the Flintstones and "th-th-that's all folks!" from Porky Pig. He didn't play American games like baseball or basketball, he didn't really care about girls or video games, and he preferred to spend his time watching TV alone or drawing. He was never invited out with friends after school or on the weekends, but that suited him just fine. He was an only child and more comfortable on his own.

School had always been pretty easy for him, once he learned enough English. He got good grades in all of his classes and never got into any trouble with the teachers. In fact, he never even got noticed by the teachers or any of the other kids. He was just there, like a silent shadow, neither liked nor hated, just ignored. Until this year.

Finally, Bhanu's name was called, and he and his father were ushered into one of the stark interview rooms within the APS. Bhanu's father held him by the elbow and guided him to the hard plastic chair where the psychiatric resident gestured for him to sit. Bhanu slumped down in the hard plastic chair and kept his eyes focused on the floor. His face was dark and glum. He looked much younger than the number 13 written on his registration sheet.

His father looked expectantly at the resident who said, "So, Mr. Patel, Bhanu, I read on the note from the triage nurse that your school insisted that you come here today. Why don't you tell me what's going on."

Bhanu remained silent. His father waited for him to talk, but his eyes remained focused on the floor. When he realized his son wouldn't speak, the father cleared his throat and said, "My son has always been good in school, but this year, something is not right, the school is giving him trouble."

Bhanu interjected softly, "It's not the school, it's the kids."

"What do you mean, Bhanu?" the doctor asked.

"Everything was fine until we had to do the groups. Eighth grade is group year. We have to do a group project in every class, to teach us team building or something. But I don't like working with the other kids," said Bhanu, with his eyes still on the floor.

"How come?" asked Dr. R.

"They make stupid jokes and call me names. They call me Poo-Poo Bhanu," he said, his face falling once again toward the floor. He thought they were slow and lazy and didn't want the other kids' work to bring down his grade. The kids thought he was a dorky nerd and didn't care if they brought down his grade.

"They are stupid anyway. I hate them all, especially Derek."

"Derek? Why?"

"He's in my science group, and he never listens to me. I was trying to tell the group about an experiment I thought we should do, but he kept interrupting. He was just trying to show off for Betsy; he has a crush on her. He kept interrupting me, and so I told him to shut his fat mouth. Then Betsy laughed out loud, because he is a little fat."

"Bhanu, you must be nice to other people," Mr. Patel said softly.

Bhanu fell silent.

"What happened after that?" asked Dr. R.

"He really didn't like me then. He did everything he could to make my life miserable. Every time the teacher turned around, he whispered something mean at me. When I walked by him in the hall, he would bump me on purpose, but make it look like an accident. One time he did it so hard, I tripped and dropped my books. And he got all of his friends to join in, too. Whenever I walked by them, they would all point at me and laugh."

Mr. Patel added, "Bhanu started getting nervous to go to school every day. He kept saying his stomach didn't feel right, or his head didn't feel right. But

I still made him go; school is the most important thing. He told me about the kids making fun of him, but I told him to ignore it, to focus on his studies."

Bhanu started hiding in the boys' bathroom during lunch, so he wouldn't have to see those kids, but Derek found him there, too.

One morning just before homeroom when the whole class was milling about waiting for the bell to ring, Derek walked up to Bhanu, who was sitting with his head slumped over his desk, and handed him a small pencil box with a picture of Elmer Fudd on it.

Derek said, "Here. Truce, OK?"

Bhanu took it, with a small smile spreading across his face. He looked at Derek and whispered, "OK, truce." He looked down at the pencil box and opened the top. Inside was a plastic bag. He lifted out the bag and saw that it was filled with dog poop. Bhanu looked over at Derek, who mouthed, "Poo-Poo Bhanu, Poo-Poo Bhanu." All of Derek's friends were watching, and they burst into laughter. Bhanu got up and ran from the room.

That was four weeks ago, and Bhanu still hadn't been back to school. Every morning when his dad came to wake him for school, he would say that he was too tired to get out of bed. The sound of those boys laughing echoed in his head and gave him a sick feeling in his stomach. He didn't have the energy to face that laughter again. He spent the whole day sleeping. He barely got up at all, barely ate a thing. His father took him to the pediatrician, who ran blood tests to see if he had mono and to check his kidneys, thyroid, and blood count; all of his tests were normal. The pediatrician told him he was probably recovering from a virus and he should just go back to school. But Bhanu still would not get out of bed.

"Can the school really take him to court? Can they do that?" asked Mr. Patel nervously.

"I think they were probably talking about a CHINS, a Child in Need of Services hearing," replied Dr. R.

A CHINS is a legal case in which a parent or a representative from a school files a petition to ask the juvenile court to help them manage a child who might be running away, refusing to obey the rules of the parents, regularly skipping school, or violating school rules. When the CHINS petition is filed with the court, the child is assigned a probation officer, who works with the family to determine the rules and services that will be put into place with the goal of changing the child's behavior. These are the so-called conditions of the CHINS.

The conditions can include anything that the probation officer feels is necessary—daily school attendance, a curfew, random drug tests, anger-management groups, and/or counseling. The child and family sign this agreement, which becomes a contract with the probation officer. If the child does not abide by the contract, he can be called before the judge, who will decide if more services or restrictions are needed or if the child needs to be removed from the parent's custody and placed in the custody of the appropriate state agency. In the CHINS petition is really an attempt to scare a child straight by bringing him before a judge and invoking the power of the legal system to ensure good behavior.

Dr. R explained, "The school is probably saying that Bhanu has missed so much school that they are thinking about filing a CHINS Truant, so the judge and probation officer will make sure he gets to school. But they are first giving you the option of getting him help to deal with whatever is keeping him out of school."

"He is sick, that's what has been keeping him out of school. He just needs more time to get better," replied Mr. Patel.

"Does the school know about Bhanu being bullied by this boy?"

Mr. Patel shook his head, "When Bhanu told me about the box with the . . . contents, I wanted to call the school, but Bhanu begged me not to. He said it would just make it worse."

Dr. R asked Mr. Patel if he would wait in the waiting room so that she could talk with Bhanu alone.

When she returned to the interview room where Bhanu was sitting, sadness seemed to have filled the entire room.

"Bhanu, you look really sad," said Dr. R.

He nodded.

"Do you feel as sad as you look?"

He nodded his head again.

"Sometimes, when kids feel really sad, they can't enjoy anything anymore, not even things that used to be really fun. Has that happened to you?"

"Yes," he said softly.

"Have you been feeling guilty, like all of this is somehow your fault?"

Another nod.

"Sometimes when kids feel really, really down, they wish that they weren't here anymore, that they could go to sleep and never wake up. Do you ever have thoughts like that?"

Bhanu sat silently.

"I know it's hard to talk about, but it's important for me to know. I want to be able to help you. Do you ever have thoughts like that?" asked Dr. R again.

"Yes," he said, so softly it was almost a whisper.

"Did you ever think about what you might do to hurt yourself?"

Bhanu shook his head no.

"Do you think you would ever actually do something to hurt yourself?" asked Dr. R.

"I don't know," he said, "if I had to go back to school . . . I don't know."

* * * * *

Bullying is not a new phenomenon, and what happened to Bhanu is surprisingly common. But the way in which many kids are being bullied is new, and significantly more destructive. Most kids have cell phones with text messaging, access to Facebook and YouTube, and some form of video chat. Bullying no longer stops at the school playground. Kids can be bullied around the clock, in their bedroom or living room, through their phones or computers. And their humiliation is no longer semiprivate, or witnessed by just a few classmates; it is easily viewed by anyone with an Internet connection.

Adolescents who are bullied, regardless of the method, are far more likely to experience depression, contemplate suicide, or harm themselves than those who are not.[1] The bullies themselves are also at increased risk for depression and attempted suicide.[2] Children who are both victims of bullies and bullies themselves, called victim-perpetrators, may have the highest rates of suicidal ideation of all.[3]

Suicide by adolescents who have been bullied has become such a common concept that it has even garnered its own term: bullycide. Bullycide made international headlines in 2010, when a 15-year-old girl who had been bullied mercilessly at her Massachusetts high school hanged herself in her home. Six students were charged with felonies related to her death, and in May 2010, one of the strictest antibullying bills in the country was signed into law. This law requires schools to implement bullying-prevention plans, including antibullying training for all teachers and staff, the creation of an antibullying curriculum, and mandatory investigation of all reports of bullying. Whether this law is successful remains to be seen.

* * * * *

For Bhanu, the antibullying legislation didn't change the fact that he was being tormented in school. His teachers, managing overcrowded classrooms where the loud and disruptive kids got the attention, hadn't noticed that he was being bullied. In fact, the school administrators had only noticed Bhanu's absences and threatened to file a CHINS petition for truancy.

After a lengthy discussion, Mr. Patel accepted the idea that Bhanu's stomach problems and debilitating fatigue were not part of a physical illness but rather manifestations of a severe depression that was triggered, at least in part, by being bullied. Unfortunately, there was no way for the doctors and nurses in the APS to guarantee that Derek and his friends would no longer bully Bhanu.

But, even if Bhanu had wanted to go back to school, he wouldn't have been able to. His depression was so severe that he was no longer functioning; his mood, coupled with his social isolation and suicidal thoughts, placed him at high risk for suicide. He had no psychiatrist or therapist who could see him right away and follow him closely. Right now, he needed the safety and containment of a psychiatric hospital.

Bhanu spent two weeks as a patient on an inpatient psychiatric unit. He had intensive therapy, and due to the severity of his symptoms, he began taking an antidepressant. The treatment team also spent a great deal of time talking with representatives from his school, trying to work out a way for Bhanu to feel safe enough to return there. The school administrators had no idea that Bhanu was being bullied or that Derek was doing the bullying. Even though the teachers kept saying kids should speak up if they were being bullied, Bhanu hadn't wanted to. He thought that speaking up against Derek was what had caused his problems in the first place.

The principal called Derek's parents, investigated Derek's role in the bullying, and ultimately suspended Derek and recommended that he seek counseling. The school guidance counselor came to visit Bhanu in the hospital to see how he was doing and to encourage him to come back to school. Bhanu wanted no part of any of it.

In the end, though, Bhanu had to return to school. It's the law. As a compromise, he was allowed to do his work on his own in the resource room. Although he eventually attended for the full day, he never returned to his regular classroom, ate lunch in the cafeteria, or went outside at recess. At the end of eighth grade, his parents were thinking of homeschooling him.

Notes

1. Klomek AB, Marrocco F, Kleinman M, et al. Bullying, depression and suicidality in adolescents. *J Am Acad Child Adolesc Psychiatry* 2007 46(1): 40–49; Kim YS, Leventhal MD. Bullying and suicide: a review. *Int J Adolesc Med Health* 2008 20(2): 133–154.
2. Klomek AB, Marrocco F, Kleinman M, et al. Bullying, depression and suicidality in adolescents. *J Am Acad Child Adolesc Psychiatry* 2007 46(1): 40–49.
3. Kim YS, Leventhal MD. Bullying and suicide: A review. *Int J Adolesc Med Health* 2008 20(2): 133–154.

4

DO YOU SEE WHAT I SEE?

Amanda felt like she had been depressed since the day she was born. She was 10 years old the first time she thought about killing herself and 12 the first time she actually tried to do it by overdosing on pills she found in the medicine cabinet. Now, at the age of 15, she had already tried to kill herself three times; she couldn't even get that right.

She woke up every morning feeling a deep sadness. It stayed with her every minute of every day, making her whole body ache. She would do anything to relieve that pain. She had started cutting herself with a razor blade a few years ago—evenly spaced thin lines on her arms, thighs, and stomach. Cutting helped her feel alive for a few moments. But that feeling never lasted long enough to make a difference.

Every time she looked in the mirror, she saw a disgusting creature staring back at her. Her scraggly, mousey-brown hair hung limp, and it matched her ugly brown eyes. Her skin was pale and mottled with angry red pimples. She hated her body, the fat stomach and the fleshy thighs. She tried making herself throw up after she ate. She didn't lose that much weight, but the burn of acid in her throat that brought tears to her eyes distracted her for a little while.

After her last suicide attempt, she had been sent to an inpatient psychiatric unit near her home and then transferred to a long-term residential treatment program where she had spent the past four months. Sometimes a health insurer can be convinced to pay for this type of long-term intensive treatment, sometimes state agencies share the cost with an insurer, sometimes school districts must bear the burden, and sometimes desperate families will foot the approximately $50,000 per year the bill themselves.

But even the staff at the resi couldn't really help Amanda feel better. She went to group therapy and met with her own counselor every day, but she still felt miserable. She still wanted to cut herself, although it was much more difficult to do now than before. The staff watched her all the time and prevented her from having access to sharp objects that she could use to hurt herself. Of course, she had taken a variety of antidepressants for years. The psychiatrist who worked with all the patients living there started her on a new medication that was supposed to supplement the effect of the antidepressants and suppress her urges to hurt herself. As far as she could tell, all it did was make her body feel stiff. However, instead of stopping the new med, she had to take yet another one three times a day to treat the side effects of the first.

The past few days, she had been feeling especially broken. Her head was fuzzy, and she couldn't think right; it felt like someone had filled her brain with glue. She was so confused that she couldn't even read her favorite magazines. When she spoke with her parents on the phone, she couldn't tell them what she had been doing because she couldn't remember.

Amanda knew her parents were worried about her. They had called on Sunday to say that they were taking her to see another doctor in Boston for a second opinion, and then they showed up the next day and put her in the car.

During the ride, she began to feel even worse. Her head felt thick; her thoughts were jumbled and slow. She opened the window hoping that the air on her face would make her feel better. She couldn't understand why her sister, who was supposed to be away at college, was also in the car, and she kept trying to ask her what she was doing there. No one answered. And then she saw the bees; there were so many of them, and they were circling around her mother's head in the front seat and streaming into the back seat. No one was paying any attention. The bees were angry; they were coming toward her.

She cried, "Watch out for the bees!"

"You're imagining things, Amanda." Her mother's voice from the front seat echoed in the car, and she could see the words forming in the air in front of her as if her mother had held up a sign rather than spoken.

The next thing she knew, she was lying on a stretcher in a bare room. The lights were dim. She could see light streaming in through a glass window and people walking back and forth on the other side. She thought she still saw the bees circling in the corner of the room. She turned her head quickly to see if they were there and if they were coming toward her.

The door opened, and a young woman doctor came in. She had heard that Amanda had a history of depression, self-injurious behavior, and possibly an underlying psychosis. Her parents had brought her here for a second opinion on treatment. The triage nurse had checked her vital signs and quickly dispatched her to the APS. The APS nurse had put her in a holding room because she was only 15 and she needed to be separated from the adult patients waiting to be seen.

"Hi Amanda, I'm Dr. P, the psychiatry resident in the ED."

"The car brought me in," Amanda told her without being asked.

"Oh, right, the car. OK, why did the car or, I guess, your parents bring you in?" asked Dr. P.

"To see a doctor. I haven't been feeling well."

"What's wrong, Amanda?"

"In like sin, in like sin," said Amanda. "That rhymes. In and sin."

Amanda was making clang associations (using rhyming words that didn't really make sense in context), a behavior sometimes seen in patients who are psychotic.

Dr. P shifted gears. "Amanda, can you tell me where we are right now?"

"I'm at the doctor's. You're the proctor, doctor."

"Yes, that's right. I'm the doctor. But where are we right now?"

"The doctor's. I came to see a doctor, not a proctor."

"Where did you come from?"

"The resi."

"And how you are feeling right now?"

"Feeling? Feelings? I don't have feelings anymore. I have toes, that's all," replied Amanda, looking around the room.

"Your toes? Are your toes hurting you? Or is anything else hurting you?" asked Dr. P.

"No, there is no hurt. I feel nothing. I am nothing. No pain, no gain," replied Amanda, as she licked her lips, which seemed dry and chapped. "My dad says that." She giggled a bit.

"I'm not sure I understand," said Dr. P.

"I know, I know, no one understands me. It has been that way since the beginning, the inning, the beginning of the inning. . . ." Amanda trailed off and stared at the blank wall.

She slowly let her eyes pan the entire room as if she were standing at a great height and gazing out over a body of water or mountain range, "I know it was you, I know, I do. I know it was you who put the bees in here."

"You see bees in here?" asked Dr. P.

"Of course I see the bees. They are all over. I know you put them in here." This time, her eyes darted around the room, and she shifted restlessly on the stretcher, smacking her lips and licking them again.

"Amanda, I didn't put the bees in here. I know you see the bees, but I can't see them. Are you also hearing things that I can't hear?"

"Don't you hear the bees?"

"What kind of noises do they make?"

"Bzzzzz. Bzzzzzz." Amanda made swooping motions with her arms. "There they go. Why did you bring them here? Don't you want to help me?"

"Can I bring your parents in, Amanda?" Dr. P asked her. "Maybe they can help us with the bees."

Amanda didn't seem to hear the question at first. She glanced around the room again but then slowly nodded her head yes.

Dr. P opened the door slightly and stuck her head out so that she could get the nurse's attention. "Hey, Brian, let's bring the parents in so I can talk with them," she said. "Oh, and while you're at it, did you get her labs already? Did she pee in a cup? We need a urine tox."

"Not yet," Brian said. "I asked her if she had to pee, but she said she didn't. I did get her labs, though."

Both of Amanda's parents hurried in when summoned from the waiting room. The words tumbled out of Mrs. M. "Something is very wrong. She hasn't been doing well at the residential. We decided to bring her here to get a second opinion. Then, when we were in the car, she started seeing bees and talking to herself! She's had depression, bad depression, but she has never been like this before."

"We even had to pull over to check the whole car, but there were no bees," Mr. M added.

Dr. P ran through the differential diagnosis in her head. Sometimes kids who were extremely depressed developed hallucinations. But it would be unusual for hallucinations from depression to start so suddenly and to be so severe. No one was saying that Amanda couldn't sleep or that she had too much energy or that she had been talking very fast. Didn't sound like her psychotic symptoms were part of a manic episode.

Hallucinations can be part of a medical illness.

"Has Amanda been sick at all? Cold, flu, sore throat?" Dr. P asked.

"She's been saying her head is thick, but she was checked out by the nurse and she didn't have a fever or anything."

"Has she ever had a seizure? Or a head injury? Problems with her thyroid?" asked Dr. P.

"No, other than her depression, she has always been a healthy girl. She's cut herself, but she's never even broken a bone."

Dr. P kept running through the differential in her head. "Recreational drugs like acid (LSD) or ecstasy (methylenedioxymethamphetamine or MDMA) can make people see things that aren't there. Even marijuana can do that. Could Amanda have experimented with those?"

Mrs. M shook her head. "No, that's one thing Amanda hasn't gotten into, thank goodness. I guess one of the kids could have smuggled something in to the residential, but the staff searches them."

"How about over-the-counter stuff like cough syrup or cold tablets? Kids sometimes take those drugs because they contain dextromethorphan, which in high enough doses can produce hallucinations."

But Amanda had never taken any of those over-the-counter medications, either.

Amanda was clearly psychotic—she was hearing and seeing things that weren't there. She was awake and oriented, as she seemed to know where she was and knew that she had come with her parents from a residential facility to see another doctor, but other than that, she wasn't making a whole lot of sense. Dr. P wasn't sure what was causing the hallucinations. But at least she could treat them.

Dr. P turned to the parents. "I want to give Amanda some medication to stop the hallucinations. Has she ever taken an antipsychotic medication before?"

Mrs. M nodded. "Yes, that was the one they just started her on last week, an antipsychotic. They said it was a low dose that when added to the antidepressant, would help her depression. But she had a bad reaction to that."

"What kind of a reaction?"

"All the doctor told us was that her neck felt stiff."

"Then what happened?"

"He gave another medicine and her neck felt better."

It sounded like the antipsychotic medication had precipitated a dystonic reaction in which the muscles in Amanda's neck contracted involuntarily and went into spasm. These painful muscle contractions had resulted from an imbalance between the neurotransmitters dopamine (DA) and acetylcholine (ACH): the antipsychotic medication blocked a subset of DA receptors, which in turn led to more cholinergic activity and disrupted the delicate balance between the two neurotransmitters. The psychiatrist at the residential facility had then added another medication, benztropine, which is anticholinergic, to treat the spasms, no doubt thinking that he couldn't discontinue the antipsychotic because Amanda remained so depressed and self-injurious despite treatment with an antidepressant. Perhaps Amanda's depression had gotten much more severe; perhaps her hallucinations had been present for a while, but the parents hadn't known that.

Dr. P was worried about the psychotic symptoms. They were frightening for Amanda and for her parents. She needed to speak with the psychiatrist at the residential treatment center to find out what Amanda had looked like before she got into her parents' car. Had her mental status changed acutely? In the meantime, she decided to give another dose of an antipsychotic medication plus another dose of the anticholinergic medication to prevent the dystonia. The nurse brought in two pills a short time later, and Amanda took them with a small amount of water.

"Let's see how she does with this," Dr. P told the parents. "It's scary for her to be seeing bees when there aren't any bees. Let's try to make her feel less afraid."

Several hours went by, and Dr. P attended to other patients. She put in a call to the resi, but the psychiatrist wasn't immediately available. She left a message for him to call her back. She checked Amanda's labs; they were all completely normal. She noticed that there was still no urine tox screen in the system, so apparently Amanda hadn't peed yet. She was writing up her notes when Brian came to find her in the back room.

"Doc, you should see this kid. Something isn't right," he said with urgency in his voice.

Dr. P walked quickly into the room. Mrs. M was sitting on the stretcher holding Amanda's hand. Mr. M was standing against the wall. Amanda appeared quite flushed. Her eyes had a far-off, glazed stare.

"That medicine didn't make her any better. She actually seems worse," said Mrs. M. "She keeps talking about the bees, and she keeps trying to grab them out of the air."

"I thought you said this medication would help her," said Mr. M. He started pacing up and down the room. "Now she's just talking crazy."

Dr. P looked at Amanda. "Amanda, how are you feeling?"

"The time is now, now is the time. Time, lime, I'm . . ." said Amanda, looking at the wall. "I need to make the bed now."

She let go of her mother's hand, picked up a glass of ginger ale that had been placed on the floor by her stretcher, and started to pour it onto the sheets.

The three adults in the room watched her but did not intervene.

Finally her father said, "Amanda, honey, don't make a mess."

Amanda looked at her father, stood up, and smiled a strange, eerie smile. She got off the stretcher and started to walk toward him, but she was off balance and trying to look in all directions at once. As he put out his hands to her, she veered and walked directly into the wall.

"Whoa, Amanda, come lie down," Dr. P guided her back to the stretcher. She walked quickly to the door of the room, opened it, and called out, "Brian, I need your help. We have to get Amanda back on the stretcher, and I think we need another set of vitals."

They easily settled her back onto the stretcher as she offered no resistance but giggled softly and rubbed her forehead where she had bumped into the wall.

Brian checked her vital signs. "Temperature's up to 101 Fahrenheit and heart rate has shot up to 120," he said.

Dr. P took a closer look at Amanda's face. "Open your eyes, Amanda," she said. Amanda slowly complied. Her pupils were wide as she stared up at the doctor.

Mr. M hovered behind Dr. P. "What is going on? What is happening to my daughter?"

"She's not psychotic, she's delirious," Dr. P told him.

* * *

Delirium is a syndrome characterized by acute onset of attention deficits, disorientation and confusion, and fluctuating symptoms. Delirious patients can be organized and coherent at one moment, yet become disorganized and incoherent a short time later. Delirium can be due to a variety of causes, including, among others, infections, problems within the brain like strokes or tumors, metabolic disturbances such as changes in sodium or calcium levels, or poisoning.

Amanda had been poisoned by the very medications the doctors were using to treat her psychiatric problems.

While at the residential facility, she had been given low dose of an antipsychotic medication to amplify the effects of her antidepressant. Presumably, the addition of the antipsychotic caused her muscle spasms. To manage the painful muscle spasms, the psychiatrist at the residential facility gave her another medication, benztropine, which blocked the ACH receptors in the brain. This anticholinergic drug usually causes minimal side effects at small doses, but it can produce delirium in large doses.

The term cholinergic refers to the action of ACH, which has a complex role in transmitting signals in the parasympathetic nervous system, which controls the rest-and-digest systems including salivation, lacrimation, urination, and defecation. It is a counterbalance to the sympathetic nervous system, which is the emergency broadcast system for the body, governing the so-called fight-or-flight responses. The balance between these two systems is best seen in their shared control of the heart. The parasympathetic system works to slow the heart, and the sympathetic system speeds it up. Drugs that have anticholinergic properties work to suppress the parasympathetic system, producing symptoms such as dry eyes and mouth, rapid heart rate, and constipation. Amanda's heart rate went up because the anticholinergic effects of the drugs she had taken blocked the parasympathetic nervous system and let the sympathetic system take over.

The symptoms of anticholinergic delirium can be remembered by using a mnemonic: blind as a bat, mad as a hatter, red as a beet, hot as a hare, dry as a bone, full as a flask. Patients with anticholinergic delirium have mydriasis, or dilated pupils, making it difficult for them to see. They have psychiatric symptoms such as hallucinations or paranoia and can seem mad as a hatter. Their flushed skin makes them appear red as a beet. They can develop fevers and seem hot as a hare. They have dry skin and mucous membranes, appearing dry as a bone, and suffer from urinary retention, thus unable to pee and full as a flask.

In retrospect, Amanda came in mad, with visual hallucinations, but it was only over time that someone recognized that she was also hot (temperature of 101 degrees F) and dry, with chapped lips and the inability to pee. Dr. P finally understood the whole picture when Amanda became flushed or red and then seemed to walk blindly into a wall.

What happened to Amanda is unfortunately all too common. It is so easy to ascribe new psychiatric symptoms to the preexisting psychiatric condition. Amanda, a physically healthy 15-year-old girl, had a history of depression, self-injurious behavior, self-induced vomiting, and three prior suicide attempts. She presented to the emergency room with new symptoms—auditory and visual hallucinations, mild paranoia, and clang associations—that suggested a developing psychotic process but one that was thought to be part and parcel of an underlying mood disorder. She had been managed by an outside psychiatrist with antipsychotic medications. Everyone from the triage nurse to the psychiatric resident was misled by her history. Dr. P's choice to ameliorate her symptoms with more antipsychotic and anticholinergic medication was understandable; it was also unfortunate.

It can be extremely difficult to make the diagnosis of delirium. As in this case, the patient's mental status can change very quickly. Sometimes Amanda's speech was coherent and her responses appropriate; at other times she appeared confused and behaved irrationally. It is easy to be fooled. The treatment for anticholinergic delirium is usually supportive. After stopping the offending agent, the patient needs hydration, monitoring, and tincture of time. In particularly severe cases, doctors might administer another drug, physostigmine, a cholinergic agent that reverses the anticholinergic effects. Drugs like physostigmine inhibit the enzyme that breaks down ACH. This makes more ACH available at nerve endings, reversing the inhibiting effects of the anticho-linergic drug.

Amanda was admitted to the Pediatric Intensive Care Unit. After three days of intravenous fluids and intensive monitoring, she began to improve. After six days, she was no longer seeing or hearing things. Her mental status finally improved to the point where she was fully awake, alert, and oriented, asking the nurses why she was in a different hospital and no longer at her residential facility.

At discharge, she told her parents that she had no memory of what had happened to her after she got into the car with them. Her parents remembered everything.

5

CORNERED AND CONTAMINATED

As the trip to India loomed, 13-year-old Nicholas began to get increasingly anxious. His parents advertised it as another family adventure, just like the trip to China last summer. That trip had gone well, but when he returned home, he couldn't quite shake the feeling that he had contracted some terrible disease while he was there. Just after landing at Boston's Logan Airport, Nicholas had begun vomiting and having diarrhea. The acute symptoms subsided within days, but, still, several months later, Nicholas did not feel much better. He was sure that his stomach problems were related to a severe underlying and as yet undiagnosed illness. No amount of reassurance from his family doctor had been enough to assuage his fears. Just last month, he had insisted on having his pediatrician order tests for blood-, air-, and parasite-borne diseases. Nothing. The doctor told him to stop worrying—he was fine.

But he knew better. There was definitely something wrong inside of him, and he didn't want whatever it was to get any worse. He knew that he needed to stay away from germs. If he came into contact with germs, he might die. Or worse, if he harbored some terrible germ and no one found it, he might infect his parents or his friends and then they might die. Germs could be anywhere. They could be on the walls of the very shower stall he used to wash. They could be on the door knobs that his friends and family turned one way or another several times a day without so much as washing their hands before they did it. Germs could lurk on his clothes, his socks, his clothes, and even his hair.

What made matters even worse, he was allergic to so many things. If he ate certain nuts or fruits, he might just get an itchy rash or he might stop breathing. Luckily, he had never actually had any kind of allergic reaction, but that was undoubtedly because he never went near any nuts or fruits in the market and he refused to allow his mother to buy any for their home. He never ate any of the foods that the doctor said might cause a problem. He made his mother carry his EpiPen with her, and he also left one at school in the nurse's office.

Now he had the almost impossible job of guarding against both food and germs. How could he possibly go with his family to India? He might catch something simply from the air. And his parents said they were going to build houses in a village that had no running water. That meant no shower for two weeks. His mother told him that he wouldn't catch anything, but then she reminded him that he had to remember to drink only bottled water and cola.

There must be something he could do. Yes. He could protect himself. He could keep himself clean. That way, he wouldn't get any germs, and he wouldn't infect anyone else. But, if he took a shower, he needed to be very careful with the body wash, shampoo, and conditioner. Maybe other people had touched the containers. He wouldn't even dream of touching the bar soap; who knows what might grow on that. He had to spend enough time washing himself so that he could be sure that all the germs went down the drain. He would use a different towel to dry each arm and leg so that no germs could travel from one limb to another. All these things took time. He was going to have to tell his parents he couldn't go to India.

* * *

When his mother told him that she was taking him to the emergency room to see a psychiatrist, he panicked.

"Why, Mom?" he asked. "What did I do? This is all because I said I couldn't go with you and Dad on your trip, right?"

"Nicholas," she said. "You've been spending three hours a day in the shower. You need help."

"I just need to get myself clean," Nicholas explained. "You know that I must have caught something when we went to China."

"But that was nine months ago. Nine. There is no way that you could still be sick from that trip. The doctor did a lot of tests that proved you didn't get sick from that trip; I think you just happened to get sick when we got home."

"I know there's something they didn't find. But, really, I'm fine."

"No. You're not fine. You spend hours in the shower, your hands are red and chapped because you wash them so often, you won't open a door because you can't touch a door knob, and last night you changed your T-shirt seven times before you came down to dinner. Once you got to the table you had to use a different fork for every course. Now you tell me you can't go on this family trip. That's it. Your father and I agree."

"OK. I know I'm anxious. I am anxious. But I'll go to the doctor, really I will. I don't need the emergency room." Nicholas started to breathe in and out rapidly. "I'm going to stop. I am." His voice quavered and he wrapped his arms around himself, tucked each hand under the opposite armpit, and started shaking.

"Nicholas. Get in the car. I have tried for the last three weeks to get you to a psychiatrist. I called your pediatrician, she gave me names—none of them have time to see you. I called the insurance company, and I got some more names, but the wait is weeks or even months long. Your doctor told me that you can get an evaluation in the emergency room. You need help and you need help now."

Thus, Mrs. E drove herself and her son Nicholas to the APS. Nicholas, wearing a long-sleeved shirt, jeans, socks, and sneakers, tucked his hands into his shirt so that his hands were not visible before he agreed to talk with the triage nurse. His mother explained that Nicholas was very anxious and needed to see a psychiatrist. The triage nurse ascertained that no one was in any acute danger and told them they needed to wait their turn. The APS waiting room was full, so the two were sent over to the pediatric section of the ED to wait. No one was using the guppy room. Mother sat in one of the chairs. Nicholas stood in the middle of the room. The young woman volunteer who had escorted the two to pediatrics asked Nicholas if he would like to sit in one of the other chairs or if he would prefer to rest on the stretcher. He did not answer her; he just remained standing. Mrs. E gazed at the walls, which were decorated with marine animals in shades of blue, green, and yellow. Nicholas stared at the floor.

The attending pediatric emergency room physician poked his head in to see if everything was all right.

"He's healthy," Mrs. E told the doctor. "He has allergies to some fruits and nuts, that's all. It's probably in the record."

"You're here to see the psychiatrist, right?"

"Yes. My son needs an evaluation."

"I'll do what I can to get this moving," he said, "then I'll be back to give him a quick physical exam." The pediatrician went to call the APS to be sure that the residents knew that Nicholas was waiting.

Dr. H took the call, checked the computer to see if there were notes about Nicholas in the electronic medical record, and then grabbed a clipboard before heading over to pediatrics. He got a brief version of the story from the pediatric resident sitting outside the guppy room.

"So the emergency is that the family wants to go to India in two weeks to save the planet?" he asked.

"That seems to be it," said the pediatric resident.

* * *

Nicholas was still standing in the middle of the room; he had crossed his arms and tucked each hand under the opposite armpit. He was slender and tall with softly curling brown hair that fell in gentle waves over his face.

"Hi, Nicholas," Dr. H said, "I'm Dr. H. I'm the psychiatry resident here this afternoon. I would just like to ask you a few questions. Can you tell me why you're here today?"

Without glancing up or looking at Dr. H, Nicholas said, "My mother brought me. She thinks I'm upset and anxious because I spend a long time in the shower. But I'm fine. I do well in school."

"That's great that school is going well. But why do you spend such a long time in the shower?"

At least 30 seconds passed before Nicholas answered, "Have to protect myself from germs. I was very sick last summer. I think I have some disease that the doctors just can't find. I know I have some kind of germ. But I can fix this."

"Sorry to hear that you were sick."

"I get good grades. I run cross country. I write for the newspaper."

"How long have you been worried about germs?"

"I told you, since I got back from China. Now they want to go to India."

"India?"

"My family. We're supposed to go build houses for poor people."

"You don't want to go?"

"I can't go. No showers. And I might get sicker while I'm there. And what if I catch something and get really sick? I might give it to somebody. I could die. Or I could make someone else die." Nicholas continued to look at the floor but became increasingly agitated as he spoke.

"What do you think would help with this problem? Do you have to go on the trip?" the resident asked.

"I should go. I want to go. It's a good thing. My family likes to do these things. But I just can't go."

"Do you think that if your parents cancelled the trip then you would feel better?"

"Maybe," he said slowly, "but I don't know." Then, "I should go," he repeated.

"Do you really think you'll infect someone else and cause his death?"

"I know it sounds crazy. I don't want to die. I don't want my parents or sisters to die. I don't want to hurt anyone. I told my mother I would stop taking such long showers. If someone would just explain what infected me when we were in China, then I would be better."

"Nicholas, why are you standing in the middle of the room?"

"Can't touch anything here. This is a hospital. Too many germs."

Mrs. E had been listening to this conversation from where she sat on a chair against the wall.

"You see," she chimed in, "Nicholas is worried about germs everywhere. He needs some medication or something. We all want to go on this trip and we have the tickets. I'm sure he'll be fine once he gets there. He was fine once we got to China. We just need a psychiatrist for him and we haven't been able to find one."

"Has Nicholas been this upset before?" the resident asked her.

"Nicholas has always been anxious about something. A few years ago he was suspicious that the light switches might be full of bacteria or something, but nothing like this," she laughed. "Now he covers his hands so when he uses doorknobs, or sometimes he just pushes the door with his shoulder or leaves the door open. But he's a really good kid. Always has been."

"Has he ever seen a psychiatrist?"

"No. And that's part of the problem. I think he needs something. Our trip is in a few weeks. I've tried to get him someone—turns out it's almost impossible. I don't know how it can be so difficult to find a child psychiatrist. We can't wait a month, or even two weeks at this point."

Dr. H excused himself and went to call his attending.

"Outpatient problem," he reported. "Kid is anxious; he's always been anxious. Probably has obsessive compulsive disorder (OCD). He's washing his hands 20 times a day and showering for hours at a time. Thinks he caught some mysterious germ in China. Now he's worried he's contaminated with something terrible and is going to take himself out and everyone else, too. Won't touch anything here. Classic. No safety issues. I think he can go home."

The attending reminded the resident to check if Nicholas had had a recent streptococcal infection, on the off chance that his OCD had worsened acutely due to a pediatric autoimmune neuropsychiatric disorder associated with streptococcal infections (PANDAS). Sometimes kids who already have a predilection to OCD can become increasingly symptomatic following a streptococcal infection; this is thought to be caused by antibodies, those proteins made by the body to deactivate certain invaders like bacteria or viruses. Theoretically, in PANDAS, the antibodies neutralize the streptococcal bacteria, but they also attack parts of the brain thought to control obsessions and compulsions as well as the involuntary and abnormal recurrent movements and/or vocalizations called tics.

"Did he have any abnormal movements? Tic disorders can go along with OCD, too."

"No. Although he was standing in the middle of the room with his arms crossed and his hands tucked under his armpits."

"But nothing that looked like a tic—head turning, eye blinking, repeated sound or word?"

"Not at all."

"Ask about strep and get a rapid strep test. Sounds like his pediatrician is within our network. You can refer him into the Child Psych Outpatient clinic for an urgent eval. He'll be seen within a week. Whoever sees him in the clinic can follow up on the PANDAS issue as well. It's a long shot."

"I'm not sure that's soon enough for this family."

"Best we can do," the attending said. "There's nothing more we can do for them today."

APRIL 9, 11 A.M.

"He's back," announced the triage resident to no one in particular. Nobody looked up from what they were doing. The nurse-practitioner asked, "One of our repeat offenders?"

The resident tried again. "The kid with the OCD who thought he'd been contaminated in China—he's back. His father is with him this time."

"Who saw that kid?" someone asked.

"I think it was H."

"Well, Dr. H isn't here today. Anybody want to see why this kid bounced back after only five days?" the attending sitting in the corner asked.

"I'll do it," said the psychology intern, a young woman studying for her PhD in clinical psychology who was completing a six-month required rotation in the APS. "I'll see him. I'm interested in OCD."

The APS was not busy, so there was no need for Nicholas to go back to the guppy room in pediatrics. He and his father had been asked to wait in the unsecured waiting room within the APS itself.

The psychology intern read the details from the last visit and also saw that Nicholas had been seen by Dr. V in the Child Psychiatry Outpatient Clinic two days earlier and been prescribed a low dose of fluoxetine, an antidepressant for his OCD. His rapid strep test had been negative, and the blood test revealed a very low antistreptolysin O (ASO or ASLO) titer, which reassured Dr. V that Nicholas had not had a recent streptococcal infection. Apparently, Nicholas was supposed to have another appointment with Dr. V later in the day but had come to the emergency room instead.

Why would Nicholas be back in the ED when he had an outpatient appointment upstairs in a few hours? The psychology intern, a petite young woman with curly dark hair held back with a headband, checked to see that an interview room was free and went out to the waiting room to get Nicholas. She had decided that she would try to talk with him without his father. Maybe there was more to this story than the kid had let on the last time when Dr. H had interviewed him in the middle of the guppy room.

No such luck.

When the psychology intern opened the door to the waiting room, she encountered Nicholas again standing in the middle of the room, this time with his arms outstretched on either side, as if he were a statue gracing a courtyard. Again, he was wearing a long-sleeved shirt that he used to cover his hands; the tails of the shirt were hanging over the waist of his pants; on his feet, he wore thick white socks and sandals. His head was bent, and he was staring at the floor. Mr. E was sitting in one of the chairs scrolling through his BlackBerry. There were no other patients waiting; the receptionist behind the Plexiglas window was carefully occupying herself with a magazine.

"Nicholas," called the psychology intern, "why don't you come with me and we'll find a place to sit and talk."

"No," said Nicholas and his clipped tone betrayed his tension. "I am not changing my position." He did not look up.

"He's afraid he was poisoned by the pill he took last night," said his father.

"I'm contaminated," Nicholas said so softly that the intern could barely hear him.

His father added, "That's why we came back to the emergency room. Nicholas wouldn't go to see the doctor in the clinic. He didn't like her. She gave him the pill he thinks contaminated him. My wife says he also spent ninety minutes this morning standing in front of his shirt drawer trying to decide which of his many T-shirts were clean enough to wear. She couldn't get him to school."

"Why are you standing in that position?" the intern asked Nicholas. He was still standing in the same place with his arms out to either side. "Don't your arms hurt?"

"It's for the best."

"Aren't you uncomfortable?" she asked again.

"I don't think it's safe to touch things. It's horrible here. I just want to go home. He made me come back."

The intern turned to Mr. E with a puzzled look.

"Frankly, I'm not sure what's going on. Maybe this does have something to do with our trip to China last summer. Nicholas's a smart boy, and he thinks that this all started when we were there. Maybe he did come into contact with something that affected his brain. And neither my wife nor I understand why that doctor he saw a few days ago just started my son on medication right away," he said. "I think he would do better with some behavioral modification techniques. I think it was too soon to jump to medication. Now he thinks he's contaminated. He won't allow his arms to touch his sides because he might infect himself."

"I know it's probably not true," Nicholas added, but so softly that the intern barely heard him.

"What did you say, Nicholas?" she asked.

"I won't take any more medication," he said in a slightly louder tone. "It didn't work anyway. I can make myself stop doing these things." He shifted slightly on his feet but kept his arms stiffly out to the side. "I ate a burrito yesterday," he added for no apparent reason.

"I read in the chart that you're allergic to some foods. Is eating a burrito a big deal?"

His father said, "He's worried that if he touches food he will contaminate it and then he won't be able to eat it. So when he forced himself to eat the burrito with his hands, it was very difficult."

"You sure you can't lower your arms just a bit and let your arm muscles rest?"

"I just want to go home," Nicholas replied.

"Well, are you willing to spend some time talking with me?"

"No." Now Nicholas was emphatic. "I'm fine."

The psychology intern turned back to Mr. E. "What do you think would be most helpful at this point?"

"I'm not sure," he said with some irritation. "We came back today because when we called Dr. V this morning to tell her that Nicholas couldn't decide which shirt to wear and that he had been standing in front of his bureau drawer for 45 minutes, she said she thought Nicholas needed to be seen urgently. But being here is just making things worse. Nicholas thinks it's dirty here. It is dirty here. Isn't there somewhere else we could go?"

"I'm sorry." The psychology intern suddenly noticed how dirty the waiting room really was. An old coffee cup sat on one of the tables, the floor was littered with old graham cracker wrappers, and the walls were a dull beige color that was once some shade of white. "I know that the waiting room is a mess. But I'm not sure we have any place that would be exactly right," she said. "Let me go check with my attending to see what we should do."

* * *

"He's got bad OCD. He needs an SSRI (antidepressant/antianxiety agent) and some cognitive behavioral therapy (CBT), but right now he needs to go into the hospital," the attending told her. "It's going to be difficult to break his delusions about germs and contamination even with medication and it's going to be very difficult to convince him to take anything."

The intern replied, "I don't think he'll agree to going inpatient. Dad just wants some behavior modification techniques. And he's still wondering if maybe Nicholas did catch something when the family was in China. That's certainly what Nicholas thinks."

"CBT is great, but he's clearly going to need more intensive care for a bit. Offer the dad the inpatient option. If they want a pediatric infectious disease (ID) consult, they can do that on the outpatient basis, later. ID will think this is ridiculous."

One of the nurses came in. "Who's the kid on the cross?" she asked.

"Nicholas," the attending answered her. "He's paralyzed with fear right now."

"Yeah, well he's probably gonna faint soon if he doesn't put his arms down. Then he'll really be afraid something's wrong."

* * *

"Nicholas, do you think you might be willing to go into a psychiatric hospital?" the psychology intern asked him as soon as she went back out to the waiting room. She sat down in one of the chairs near his father and angled her head so that she could gaze up into his face, "I think it might be almost impossible for you to stop obsessing about being contaminated and trying to keep yourself clean just using will power. Maybe you'll feel safer taking some medication if you're in the hospital."

Nicholas turned his whole body without lifting his head or lowering his arms as if he were a doll mounted on a stand. Now he faced his father. "Dad, I can't go to the hospital—hospitals are dirty, filthy places. There are so many germs here and we're already in a hospital. I'll be fine at home. I just want to learn how to think different thoughts." His voice was plaintive. After this, he seemed finally to tire of holding his arms outstretched and carefully lowered them so that they hung by his sides but did not touch his clothing. His hands, which were red and chapped but not bleeding, once again disappeared into his shirtsleeves.

"Nicholas?" his dad asked, "Would you consider being admitted to the hospital?"

Nicholas started to cry silently.

Dad turned to the psychology intern, "You heard him. Now he's crying. He can't tolerate the idea of the hospital. My wife and I will never betray his trust in us. We won't let him go into the hospital if he doesn't want to."

"Betray his trust?" said the attending when the psychology intern reported this conversation. "Betray his trust?" He shook his head dismissively. "They're too busy saving the world to worry about their own kid? What does Dad want?"

"The father says that he wants a referral to someone who will do CBT," she said.

"Where does he live? Do they need to use their insurance to pay for care? If not, we can try to find them a private doc; if yes, then we'll try to find a community clinic in their area."

The psychology intern sat down. "I know Dad won't put him in the hospital, but don't you think we could commit him against his will?" she asked.

"Who? Nicholas?"

"Yes."

"No."

"Why not? I mean, he's just standing there in the waiting room. He hasn't moved much. He finally put his arms down."

"Is he dangerous to himself?"

"Well, not really," she said this slowly as if trying to think of something that she might have missed when she was reading his chart or talking to him.

"Is he threatening anyone else?"

"Of course not." This she could be sure about.

"Is he unable to care for himself?"

"Sort of," she hesitated. "He's not really functioning at all."

"At all? You told me that he is able to eat at least a burrito; I gather he's sleeping at night, right? Despite all of his obsessions and compulsive cleaning, he somehow, at least up until now, does his schoolwork and gets good grades. No one is saying that he has been absent too many days from school, are they?"

"But he's delusional. He thinks that he was contaminated by something or someone he came in contact with in China—something he caught while he was there. He thinks the one tablet of fluoxetine he took yesterday was poisonous."

"Yes. He has some crazy ideas. But he also knows that his ideas are crazy, he just can't prevent himself from thinking them. So he can reality test."

"Do you think he'll just get better?"

"No. Not on his own. But I also don't think I can force him or his parents to do anything they don't want to do."

"So we just let him walk out of here?"

"We let him walk if he wants to."

"We haven't done anything for him."

"No, we have. We have tried to understand what he is experiencing, and we have offered him what we feel is the best choice for care. Sometimes, that's all we can do."

"But what happens if he can't even get in the car because it's too dirty? Or what happens if he goes home with an appointment for a new outpatient provider and he can't get out of the house in time to get to the appointment? Or with this kid, he might not be able to even go into a doctor's office if it's too dirty."

"Then I guess he'll be back."

* * *

The psychology intern went back out to the waiting room with the discharge papers. Nicholas and his family had private insurance but were willing to pay cash for treatment if necessary. She gave them the name of a behavioral psychologist who could do CBT and who was willing to see Nicholas within the next week or two.

"We'll have to call her ourselves to set up the appointment," Dad told the intern. "Nicholas probably can't start until we get back from India. We plan to leave in just a few days. I'm sure he'll feel well enough to go and then we can try to deal with this again when we get back."

He signed the papers quickly without reading them and then said to Nicholas, "OK. These people are no help. Let's go."

Nicholas didn't move.

"Come on, Nicholas," his dad said. "We can go home now."

Nicholas just stood silently with his head bent. It was difficult to tell if he were still crying.

"Nicholas," Dad's voice sounded impatient now.

Slowly Nicholas raised his arms again. He pivoted sideways and began to take small measured steps toward the door.

The father went on ahead. The psychology intern sat very still in her chair. Nicholas very slowly sidestepped his way through the waiting room. He paused at the door and waited for his dad to open it. Again, he stepped sideways, arms outstretched, carefully maneuvering himself through the doorway without touching the frame. As soon as he passed the threshold, the door swung shut behind them.

6

THE WHIRLING DERVISH

Managing an agitated child, particularly a very young child, makes even experienced ED doctors and nurses anxious. There's something extremely frightening about a little kid who is out of control—kicking, hitting, spitting, scratching, biting—one who does not respond to a calm, reassuring voice or a gentle hug from someone he or she knows and trusts. Even kids who throw their toys at a sibling or punch the wall or pull the dog's tail can usually be talked down or separated from others. Teenagers who storm around and cause scenes will often hide in their rooms or leave the house for a while. Most kids stop themselves before the yelling, posturing, and threats cross that line into kicks, punches, and destruction of people or property. Those who do not often end up in the ED after family members or teachers have called 911. The emergency medical technicians or paramedics who are the first responders sometimes have to muscle such kids on to the stretcher, tie them down, and drive them in to the hospital.

Kids who have rages are often both diagnostic dilemmas as well as management nightmares. In the APS, we remind ourselves that an out-of-control child could be hungry, overtired, overstimulated, or in pain. We try the common sense remedies first: we offer food, pudding, applesauce, pizza, graham crackers, juice, or ginger ale; we try to place the child in a private room with few distractions and nothing available to use as a weapon; we offer sedating medication if the child has had experience taking such pills before. Children with developmental disabilities, particularly those who have trouble with speech and language and cannot articulate what's wrong, can become aggressive and violent when their ear hurts or they have a stomachache. Without the words to describe what they are experiencing, they often lash out at those closest to them. No one likes to hold a child down, keep him in locked leather restraints so that he does not kick or hit a staff member or himself, or give him an intramuscular injection of a sedating medication when all else fails. Yet sometimes there is no alternative; the job is to keep everyone—the child, the family members, the nurses, and doctors—safe. This can be a particularly challenging task in a busy and chaotic ED setting.

The call came in from a local elementary school, and the resident who took the triage dutifully recorded in the electronic medical record what he heard from the referring school psychologist: seven-year-old girl, first grader at the Beethoven School, living with mom in East Boston, with a history of a mood disorder of some unknown type characterized by intermittent periods of out-of-control behavior and attention deficit hyperactivity disorder (ADHD). Her mother had sole custody as her father was in jail for a drug-related crime. Her psychiatrist prescribed valproic acid (Depakote, an antiepileptic drug used by psychiatrists as a mood stabilizer) to regulate her mood and clonidine (a medicine often used to control blood pressure) for the impulsivity and distractibility characteristic of ADHD. She had had no prior hospitalizations, and her mother was driving her to the ED after the school nurse had called to report that Jasmine had been demonstrating increasingly aggressive behavior and threatening to kill other kids at school. Specifically, she had said that she would stab a classmate with a pencil. The school administrators and teachers were also concerned because over the last few weeks Jasmine occasionally zoned out. More recently she had started running out of the classroom and even out of the school building unexpectedly. The last three times this had happened, the staff had been unable to catch her before she reached the busy street.

A quick computer biopsy yielded the helpful information that Jasmine already had an outpatient child psychiatrist and had had a fairly recent evaluation by a pediatric neurologist due to an episode of apparent unresponsiveness. The diagnosis of epilepsy had been entertained but subsequently ruled out with a normal electroencephalogram (EEG), so it seemed that these episodes of zoning out were probably not seizures. She had been removed from the mainstream class in her elementary school several months earlier and placed in a behaviorally-based therapeutic classroom after she impulsively punched one of the other first graders in the face. Neuropsychological testing to clarify her learning style had been scheduled for later in the month. Someone had entertained the idea that her impulsive outbursts of aggression might stem from frustration at her inability to learn. Her outpatient doctor was in the process of adjusting Jasmine's medications. The consensus among those residents sitting and chatting in the back room of the APS was that Jasmine would most likely need an inpatient hospitalization to allow for further diagnostic assessment, to determine the cause of her recent escalation in behavior, and to tune up her psychiatric medications. Such an admission might also expedite the neuropsychological testing; the usual wait could be as long as several months. To the assembled staff, Jasmine seemed like a standard case for a Thursday afternoon and not such a tough one at that. She had not been so out of control that the school had had to call the paramedics. This seemed like an improvement from the last time she became angry and threatening. The fact that she was able to come in willingly with her mother was a good sign. She had not chosen today to run out of the school and into the street. Not much to do except talk with her, feed her, call her outpatient providers, obtain insurance approval, and find her an inpatient bed somewhere in the system.

Enter Jasmine, age seven.

She and her mother, Ms. H, walked in holding hands. They were met by the triage nurse who measured Jasmine's pulse, blood pressure, respiratory rate, and temperature. These vital signs were within normal limits. A psychiatry resident whose job was to decide where Jasmine should wait until someone had time to evaluate her came to the triage desk. Jasmine was sitting quietly, but because the school psychologist who referred her had mentioned her tendency to wander away and her recent threat to stab a classmate with a pencil, the resident thought it safest to place Jasmine in one of the holding rooms on a Section 12 within the locked section of the APS. The Section 12, also known as a pink paper because of the actual color of the paper on which it is printed, is a commitment paper. It allows health care providers to detain a patient against his or her will on the basis of dangerousness to self, dangerousness to others, or inability to care for himself or herself. With the Section 12 in place, even though Jasmine's mother had legal custody, she would not be able to take Jasmine out of the ED before the child had been fully evaluated and a safe disposition had been found. Also, once in a holding room, Jasmine wouldn't be able to roam around the rest of the ED, which was full of other patients in various degrees of distress. There wasn't much in the holding room except a stretcher, and it was certainly not possible to wander away under the watchful eyes of the security guards and nurses who sat within three feet of one of the doors. While Jasmine was in triage, another member of the team had paged the child psychiatry resident to give him a heads-up when Jasmine came through the door.

Jasmine came along quietly. Her mother followed. They walked single file behind the security guard; another guard brought up the rear. Jasmine was sniffling just a little bit and wiping her runny nose with her hand. She looked pale and small, especially compared to her mother, who was quite heavyset and imposing even in her purple T-shirt, black shorts, and flip-flops. Jasmine's reddish hair was cut short with bangs. Her sneakers were dirty and untied. Threading their way past the receptionist and the desk where the nurses sat, the two entered Bay 41, the middle room in a line of three private holding rooms usually reserved for children or for adult patients who were too intoxicated or agitated to be managed safely elsewhere.

"Why are you putting Jasmine in here?" were the first words from the mother as Sarah, the nurse, entered the room behind them and asked Jasmine to hop up on the stretcher and change into some hospital PJs. The PJs consisted of a loose top with snaps in the back and a pair of pants, and Sarah put them down on the stretcher next to Jasmine. Both the top and the pants were covered with mini but colorful teddy bears. Mindful that young children are often irritable when hungry, Sarah had some saltines in her hand in case Jasmine was hungry and wanted a snack.

"My daughter didn't do anything wrong; she doesn't need to be locked up. We are here to talk with a doctor about why she is having such trouble at school. Maybe she just needs a new medication." The mother's voice got louder as she talked until she was practically yelling by the time she got to the word medication.

No one got a chance to explain to the mother that the staff felt that Jasmine needed the privacy and safety of the holding room in order to prevent her from running away and to protect her from witnessing what was happening in other parts of the ED. With no warning, Jasmine threw the PJs on the floor, leaped off the stretcher, and ran for the door. Caught mid-stride by the nurse, who dropped the packages of crackers as she went for her, Jasmine spun around and lunged again for the door just as the child psychiatry resident, Dr. L, walked in. Dr. L instinctively headed for the opposite corner of the room. Immediately, Jasmine went for Dr. L. She began kicking at his legs, tried to grab the hospital identification badge that was clipped to his shirt pocket, and then to lift his beeper and phone from his belt. Dr. L was thrown off guard and not sure what to do. He quickly backed out the door as Jasmine pranced around him placing well-aimed kicks at his shins. The two security guards who had been sitting right outside the door went in to take control of the situation. These two men looked like members of the secret service in their blue sports coats, gray slacks, black shoes and radio earpieces. They were large, powerful, and very experienced with agitated patients, kids, or adults. Generally, the sight of Michael, who stood six feet tall and weighed 200 lbs and who spoke short, declarative sentences in a soft voice, calmed a kid right down. No such luck this time; soothing words had no effect. One guard tried to catch Jasmine's arm in order to redirect her, but she had started punching the wall with her fists.

"Don't you touch her," screamed her mother. "Get your hands off of her." When nothing happened, she yelled, "I said take your hands off my child!"

The other security guard turned to the mother and asked her to leave the room in order to give Jasmine a chance to calm down. "I'm sorry, Ma'am, but you'll have to step out now and wait for your daughter in the waiting room," he told her. "We'll help Jasmine. She's safe here." He gently took her by the arm to escort her out, telling Sarah, as he did so, to take the stretcher out of the room and leave the mattress on the floor.

"Get your stinkin' hands off of me," Ms. H demanded. "Nobody takes me away from my child." But, despite her words, she went quietly with the man in the blue sports coat as Jasmine began yelling "No, no" and crying, first flailing her arms and legs and then, as the mattress hit the floor and the stretcher was pulled out through another door, holding on to the leg of the stretcher and allowing herself to be dragged along the floor.

Such a temper tantrum, particularly in a young girl, attracted the attention of much of the unit staff, and one of the security guards called for backup. Michael pried Jasmine's hands off the stretcher bars. Jasmine began head-butting him. The security guard did the best he could to protect Jasmine from hurting herself, but when he let go of her arms, the girl threw herself to the ground and began banging her head on the tile floor.

Sarah hovered in the background, "Now, now, Jasmine, time to settle down. Listen to me, Jasmine, time to settle down." Her words had absolutely no effect.

"Where is the doc; we need the doc," Michael told her.

She called down the hallway to the work room where Dr. L had retreated to call his attending. He had never been assaulted by a seven-year-old and he didn't know exactly what to do. "Can you come back here? I think Jasmine's going to need a little something to get her to calm down and stop trying to hurt herself," Sarah was insistent.

Dr. L walked back down the hallway and stood outside Bay 41. He hesitated. "Do we know if she takes medication at home?" he asked. "Where is her mother? We can ask her."

"Yeah, valproate and clonidine, was what I heard in report from triage," answered Sarah. "And security put the mother in the waiting room last I heard."

"Did you offer Jasmine something already?"

"Look at her. Does she look like the kind of kid who's ready for a PO (*per os*—by mouth) med?" Sarah retorted.

"Well, we have to offer her something by mouth first. We can't just give her a shot. Let's give her an extra dose of clonidine. And it would be helpful to let her mother know what we're doing."

"Jasmine, Jasmine, listen to me. Will you take a medicine like you do at home? It will help you relax. If you take a dose of clonidine, you'll feel better." Sarah spoke with the tone of someone who was sure her words were in vain.

"I already had my medicine today. Get away from me," Jasmine cried, throwing herself to the floor once more and curling up into a ball.

"Let's just try, Jasmine, I can give you some to drink—you won't even have to swallow a pill." Sarah bent down to put her hand on her shoulder, and Jasmine spit at her. "No medicine, no medicine, no medicine." She rolled away, got to her feet, and began running around the room. She spied the crackers on the floor and seized one of the packages.

Allison, the nurse clinician who had been trained in how to place kids in a therapeutic hold, had been watching the drama unfold. Now she had had enough. She marched down the hallway to Bay 41, went in, and approached Jasmine from behind, hooking her arms around her chest, and sat down on the floor. Jasmine kicked her feet and struggled, twisting and turning with such force that Allison had to let go. Jasmine dropped the package of crackers and began grinding it with her foot. She picked up the cracker crumbs and started throwing handfuls of them at the staff.

"We need an IM (intramuscular injection)," Allison said to Sarah and Michael. "This isn't going to work any other way. And it seems like she's already started spitting. Don't know what that resident is thinking."

"No medicine," Jasmine started yelling again. Then her voice became a high-pitched scream, "Mom, mom, mom." She was now running around the small room, shoe laces flapping, slipping on the cracker crumbs as she went.

Dr. L returned. "I can't find the mother in the waiting room to ask her. Don't know where she went, she just left. My attending says that we can give her 12.5 mg of IM diphenhydramine. It should be plenty sedating."

Given the green light, four adults converged on Jasmine—two security guards, Allison the nurse clinician, and a nursing assistant. They placed her as gently as possible on the mattress that was still in on the floor in the middle of the room and each staff member held a different limb. Sarah went to the medicine cabinet and drew up the diphenhydramine into the syringe. Jasmine continued screaming, "Help me, help me somebody, somebody help me!"

The receptionist came around the corner. "The mother came back, heard Jasmine screaming, and is now demanding to come back in," she told Sarah.

"Tell her she can't come back until we get that child settled down. That's just the way it is," and Sarah hustled off to give Jasmine her injection.

"But she's threatening to call the police."

"Whatever," Sarah said.

Jasmine was still screaming at the top of her lungs. "No medicine, no medicine. Mom, mom, mom." Her voice echoed in the empty room.

"I'm going to give you a shot to help you calm down," Sarah told her as she took hold of Jasmine's left arm and quickly administered the shot. "There, there," she added. "That wasn't too bad, was it? You'll feel better soon."

The other four continued to hold Jasmine down on the mattress. She was sweaty and trembling, and her T-shirt was twisted around her torso. Two more security guards wheeled the stretcher frame back into the room, and those holding Jasmine carefully lifted her and the mattress up and slid the mattress back onto the metal frame. Then they placed each of Jasmine's hands and feet in soft bandage-like restraints, and tied each one to a sidebar.

"Just a few more minutes and we'll let you out of these," Allison told her. "Take a deep breath, try to relax."

Jasmine started crying and hiccupping. Twenty minutes went by. The nursing assistant sat in a chair near her head and talked to her in a low voice. Jasmine's eyelids started to droop.

"Okay. Let's let her out of those restraints. Looks like the med tired her out," Dr. L told them as he entered the room and approached her. "Hi, Jasmine, I'm Dr. L. Can you talk with me? Let's get you untied and maybe you'll sit up and talk with me?"

"Dr. L, Dr. L," Sarah poked her head into the door. "The police are here and they are asking to speak with you."

"The police?"

"Yeah. Jasmine's mom heard her crying and demanded to be let in immediately. When security told her that couldn't happen, she said she was going to call the police."

"She called the police?" Dr. L repeated in an unbelieving tone.

"That's what I'm telling you." Sarah didn't waste words.

Jasmine continued crying. She tried to straighten out her T-shirt. She pulled at her shorts. She wouldn't look up at the resident. She grabbed her left arm with her right hand and rubbed it. "You hurt me," she muttered, followed by "I'm hungry."

"Well at least the diphenhydramine worked a bit," Dr. L said basically to himself as he left again to find out what the police wanted.

"Let's get you cleaned up and into some clean, dry clothes," offered the nursing assistant, "then your mom can come in and we'll get you something to eat."

"French fries. I want French fries, French fries, French fries," Jasmine's voice was now singsong, and her demand became almost a chant.

"You settle down and we'll bring you some French fries," Allison told her. "Show us you can be in control."

The APS staff has the ability to order food for children in the ED from the hospital's main cafeteria. Sarah called the order down and asked that it be sent up as soon as possible.

"With ketchup," Jasmine added.

"Sure. Ketchup, too. But you need to change out of those clothes."

Jasmine sat quietly. She was able to accept some help getting her clothes changed. The PJs with the teddy bears on them were too big for her, and the pants dragged on the floor. The French fries arrived on a tray with several packages of ketchup, and soon she sat on the floor dipping each one carefully into a small pile of ketchup before putting it in her mouth. Her mother came in, and Jasmine barely looked up. Mother was irate and waving her arms.

She hugged Jasmine to her, saying, "I would never have done what they did to you. I want you to know I've called the police." She turned to the staff members still in the room, "I don't care about any of your opinions after what you just did to my daughter."

"Mrs. H," Sarah poked her head in, "the police have arrived, they spoke with the doctor, and now they want to talk with you."

"I will not be separated from my child again. You can have them come back in here and I'll talk with them or you can escort me and Jasmine out to speak with them," she insisted.

"We can't allow the policemen in the APS because they carry guns—that's against hospital policy," Sarah explained. "And we can't allow Jasmine to leave the unit right now. Would you like to talk with them outside?"

"I refuse to leave this room," Mother raised her voice again. "I refuse to leave my child to you people. I don't trust any of you. You have been abusing her. I want her transferred to another hospital. I want her transferred now!"

"I wasn't abused." Jasmine spoke with her mouth full as she continued to munch on her French fries.

Michael, the security guard, came back into the room and stood politely with his arms at his sides. "Ma'am," he said in a voice that brooked little argument, "you dialed 911 and reported that your child was being abused by the doctors at the MGH. The police are here now and they need to speak with you. I can't let them into this special part of the ED. Would you be able to talk with them if I brought them right to the back door of this room that opens to another part of the ED?"

"Fine," Mother said. She moved over to stand near the opposite doorway, turning her back on Jasmine while the policeman explained to her that Jasmine was in the APS on a Section 12, a commitment paper that allowed the doctors and nurses to evaluate and manage her as necessary in order to keep her and others safe.

"The doctors and nurses have a right to keep your daughter here until they feel she is safe to leave," he informed her.

"Well, then I want her transferred to another ED," Mother insisted. "These people are out to get her."

Jasmine chose that moment to escalate. She started throwing ketchup-covered French fries into the far corners of the room. She took the small ketchup packages that the nursing assistant had opened for her and began dripping the ketchup on the floor. She flung the empty packets at her mother. She squatted, put her hands in the ketchup, and then stood up and rubbed them on her cheeks and up and down her legs. Dipping her hands in the ketchup still left on her tray, she ran fast and forcefully at the wall, as if she were trying to break it down and push her way out into freedom. The air in the room grew dense with the sickly sweet smell of ketchup.

Security rushed in, crushing French fries underfoot as they moved. The police left, closing the outside door behind them. Mother turned around and raised her hand as if getting ready to hit Jasmine. The staff gathered again. Once more Jasmine started screaming, "No medicine, no medicine, no medicine." Round two had begun.

* * *

Handling an agitated child in an ED is not like running a code on an unresponsive patient in cardiac or respiratory arrest. There is no algorithm but rather the need for a certain amount of flexibility and finesse. Sometimes we can distract even a four-star temper tantrum with containment and French fries; sometimes the child bolts for the door and those French fries end up becoming ammunition rather than nourishment. Sometimes evaluation and management becomes seclusion and restraint and can look to an untrained eye like abuse and neglect, particularly when, as in this case, the evaluation and management involve what is euphemistically referred to as mechanical restraint.

Always, we must be guided by the need for safety. We must do what is in the best interest of the youngster and keep her safe from self-injury and others safe from her. The out-of-control or raging young child can be surprisingly dangerous and destructive. Jasmine was only a little girl, but she proved to be quite a match even for the experienced staff in the APS. There are few guidelines for how to manage a child like Jasmine, who suffers from affective dysregulation—another way of saying intermittently explosive and aggressive behavior. In one study, nearly 7 percent of pediatric patients (5–18 years) who presented to an ED with psychiatric problems required restraints.[1] But despite the high incidence, there are no standardized recommendations for management.

In Jasmine's case, the resident knew enough about her to place her in a holding room at the outset. Jasmine's history of unpredictable aggression toward her classmates and elopement from school was enough to justify containment and legal restriction to the unit under a Section 12 for further evaluation. But, as it turns out, simple containment was not enough. Jasmine quickly became aggressive, putting herself and others in the room at risk for injury.

Sometimes, the presence of a soothing parent, an empathic caregiver, or even a "show of force" from the security guards, can help a youngster to settle down. Not in this case. In fact, Jasmine's mother was angry and provocative; few parents call 911 from their cell phones to report that a loved one is being abused by the physicians in an ED. Even when she was with Jasmine, she was loud, demanding, inappropriate, and eventually, potentially violent herself.

As for Mother's insistence that we transfer Jasmine to another ED? Not possible in the short term. The Emergency Medical Treatment and Labor Act (EMTALA), enacted by Congress in 1986, requires that patients in EDs be stabilized before transfer. If Jasmine had calmed down and was able to maintain good behavior, her mother could request in writing a transfer to another hospital. However, the receiving hospital would have to be willing to accept Jasmine in transfer. As few EDs are well equipped to handle agitated children, it would have been extremely difficult to find one that would take Jasmine under these circumstances.

Ideally, Jasmine would have accepted a familiar sedating medication that she takes at home, but she was too upset and oppositional to do that. Perhaps, her mother used medication to quiet her down when things got out of control at home, perhaps not; whatever the reason, Jasmine was not willing to negotiate. At a certain point, Jasmine left the staff with little choice but to use IM medication to quiet her.

The question of which medication to choose for a patient like Jasmine also has no definitive answer. Even though others on the staff were irritated with his measured stance, believing that Jasmine required an IM injection, Dr. L's choice of first offering a PO med was appropriate. He chose clonidine because Jasmine took it at home. He could have also chosen a small dose of one of the atypical antipsychotic medications such as risperidone or olanzapine that are often used to manage emotional outbursts. Risperidone comes in a liquid form and olanzapine in tablets that dissolve under the tongue—both possible for a young child to manage. He probably chose the clonidine because Jasmine's mother had left, and he couldn't inform her that he was giving Jasmine a new medication, possibly one she had never tried before. Given the urgency of the situation, he did not have to tell the mother what he was doing, but his goals of trying to keep her informed and part of the process were understandable. His choice of IM medication was also reasonable, although it is true that some kids will have a paradoxical response to diphenhydramine and become increasingly hyperactive rather than lethargic.

Did Jasmine have such a paradoxical response? It's difficult to know. She appeared sleepy following her first injection, but then after 20 minutes or so, her behavior worsened acutely. Was it the diphenhydramine that caused her to escalate the second time or was it that she just hadn't gotten a large enough dose on the first go-round to keep her drowsy?

* * *

So what happened to Jasmine, still there in the holding room, now bloodied with ketchup? Sarah, a psychiatric nurse with decades of experience, took it on herself to fix the problem.

"Everyone out," she ordered. "It's a wrap," she told security. "We go to locked leathers; no more soft restraints. Get Dr. L over here again. I'm going to need an order."

Next thing Jasmine knew, four security guards materialized. They hoisted her back on to the stretcher and secured each limb in a leather strap and buckled the strap to the frame of the stretcher. Within minutes, Jasmine stopped struggling and lay quietly on the mattress.

The two security guards, Sarah, and the nursing assistant stayed with her. They spoke to her quietly, saying that if she stayed calm for a bit, they would free one of her arms and one of her legs, let her sit up and have a drink through a straw. She did well and was coaxed into taking a dose of liquid risperidone, which tired her out but did not put her to sleep. Time passed. Jasmine continued to lie quietly. The security guards gradually took her out of the remaining restraints. One of the nursing assistants wiped Jasmine's face and hands, gave her a pillow, and tucked a cotton blanket around her. Eventually, she slept.

Seven hours later, Jasmine was transferred without incident to an inpatient psychiatric facility with her mother's consent.

Note

1. Dorman DH, Mehta SD. Restraint use for psychiatric patients in the pediatric emergency department. *Pediatr Emerg Care* 2006 22(1): 7–12.

7

THE ASTRONOMER

New Year's Eve 2004. Even though it was early in the evening, the ED was already hopping. Boston's First Night festivities on the Esplanade provided a steady stream of revelers. A man burned his hand shooting off fireworks from his balcony; a drunk driver crashed his car into a street sign; a woman developed an allergic reaction to her glitter body paint and was rushed to a cubicle in Acute. The APS was no different; already every room was filled. In Bay 40, a prisoner who had tried to hang himself in his cell. In Bay 41, a homeless woman who chased a group of tourists down the street threatening to kill them and who continued to hurl expletives at the staff. In the waiting room sat an elderly man who stumbled into the APS intoxicated and suicidal with a plan to throw himself in front of a train; a middle-aged woman comforted her sister who was sobbing and drumming her feet; an anorexic young woman who voiced a chief complaint of anxiety and was dressed in many layers of outerwear sat quietly staring off into space.

Fifteen-year-old Austin and his mother, a matched pair with fair skin, freckles, and coarse red hair walked into the ED about 7 P.M. They were wearing parkas, hats, and mittens, having walked to MGH through the icy slush and biting wind, all at Austin's insistence.

Even though they had been at the homeless shelter only a few days, he couldn't stand another minute there—the air was thick and felt saturated with germs, every surface had years of dirt ground into it, and even the tap water tasted unclean. Furthermore, his schedule kept getting interrupted; he couldn't shower at the time he always did at home, he couldn't have his meals at exactly the time he was used to, and he couldn't even go to sleep at his proper bedtime because people kept waking him up. Austin needed to keep to his schedules and routines; they helped him to remain calm and settled. When his routines were interrupted, his muscles started to tense, and he got so anxious he couldn't think straight. First he became irritable and weepy, then angry and desperate.

Austin had Asperger's disorder, which lies on the mild end of the autism spectrum. Kids with Asperger's have significant trouble with social interactions;

they have a hard time reading social cues, and they often express themselves in an odd, pedantic manner. Because they struggle both to understand their peers and to make themselves understood, it can be difficult for them to make friends and easy for them to become the targets of bullies. They thrive with consistency and predictability, and when their routine is interrupted, they struggle to adapt. These children often show intense interest in a specific subject, and this interest can become all-encompassing. They will spend hours a day learning about (and talking about) one particular subject such as the history of ski lifts in North America, or the biology of starfish, or the names of every star in the sky.

Before they arrived in Boston, Austin and his mother had been living in a neighboring state, in a farmhouse his uncle owned. They had lived there for three years, since the day his mother left his father and his father disappeared. Her brother had taken them in and let them live rent-free. It wasn't perfect, but it worked. At the farmhouse, each day was predictable. Austin got up in the morning and boarded the bus to the high school. His special class met in one room; there he could work at his own pace. The kids knew him and had grown used to his odd ways; they no longer teased or taunted him. In his uncle's house, Austin had his own room where he kept his collection of astronomy books. He had mounted an old telescope on the back porch, and he would spend hours outside studying the night sky. He knew hundreds of the stars by name as well as their distance from earth, their magnitude, and their spectral type. He loved to think about the stars, to make lists of them in his mind, and to arrange them by size, distance, or magnitude. He could talk about the stars forever, and he would, with anyone who would listen.

Then one night in late December, his mother argued with his uncle. The two yelled and shouted and blamed the other one for their problems. Before Austin knew it, his mother told him to pack quickly and fit everything into one bag. Later that night, they got on a bus to Boston. When they got off at South Station, they had no place to stay, hardly any money, and no plan. His mother found her way to a homeless shelter and told Austin they would be there for a very short time. Austin had had to get ready so fast that he had left his telescope behind.

After a day or two, a social worker came by the shelter and met with him and his mother. She reminded them that Austin needed to enroll in one of the Boston public schools. He asked her about special classrooms like the one he had been in at home—did they have those here, too? Maybe, she told him, but he couldn't start in one right away; his mother would have to request it, and there would be tests and then meetings. It could take weeks or even months. Austin felt like crying.

Today, he had spent the whole day worrying about the new school he was supposed to start in a few days, the kids and teachers there, and the shelter where nothing was clean enough. He got himself so unsettled that he could do nothing else but worry and pace. At home, when he was upset, he would go outside to his telescope. When he focused on the stars, his mind would slow down, and his whole body would relax. He would say the names of the stars out loud and recite their size and distance from the earth. He felt reassured and contained by hearing the sound of his own voice counting the stars.

Tonight, he had left the shelter, hoping that, even without his telescope, he could see the stars from the street outside. But the ambient light blocked his view of the night sky. People jostled him as he stood on the sidewalk, head tilted, straining to see something. Strangers, many already drunk, hurried past, not watching where they were going as they headed to First Night.

Austin tried to remain very still and turn his gaze upward. Someone bumped into him from the side; taken by surprise, he fell to the ground, catching himself on his outstretched arm and jamming his shoulder. It hurt, his whole body hurt, on the inside and out. He had had enough. He went inside and demanded that his mother take him to see a doctor. He was firm, even stubborn, and when he raised his voice and started to tremble, his mother gave in.

And so here they were on New Year's Eve at the MGH ED. The nurse registered Austin, and then he and his mother waited in the crowded main waiting room. They sat for hours, as more and more people straggled in. His mother tried to convince him to leave several times, but he was insistent; he would not go back to the shelter until he saw a doctor about his shoulder. At some point, his mother became engrossed in watching the Boston Pops Orchestra playing on TV and stopped pestering him to leave. When the nurse finally called his name around 2 A.M., his mother was asleep in her chair, so he went alone with the nurse into the examining room in Fast Track, the part of the emergency room reserved for people who presumably have something wrong that is easily managed in a short period of time. It was so late that the pediatrics section of the ED had long since closed; all patients, regardless of age, ended up in the same place. Austin sat down on the gurney and looked around. The room smelled of antiseptic and bleach, harsh but clean. The starched scratchy hospital sheet was rough against his hands. The counters in the room were freshly wiped, without a trace of dust. The shelves had labels, and each item was in its place. It was clean and orderly here. His eyes began to well up with tears.

The doctor entered the room; he was brusque and efficient. He asked Austin how he had hurt himself, and Austin told him about being bumped and falling. He explained that he had used his outstretched arm to break his fall and that now his shoulder hurt a lot. The doctor began to feel Austin's shoulder. He asked him to show him where it hurt and which movements made it better or worse. As he tried to do what the doctor asked him, Austin started to cry. Once he started, he just couldn't stop.

The doctor finished examining Austin's arm and told him he hadn't broken anything. But still Austin cried. The doctor told him that the injury was so minor that he didn't even need an X-ray. But still Austin cried. The doctor got nervous, unsure what to do with a fifteen-year-old who just wouldn't stop crying. He asked Austin if he would like his mother to come in. Austin nodded yes through his tears, and one of the nurses went to wake her up. But, even with his mother there, he couldn't stop his tears. The doctor explained to Austin's mother that Austin's shoulder was fine. His mother told the doctor that Austin had Asperger's and that they had recently moved to Boston. She sat down heavily on one of the chairs in the room and put her head in her hands. Austin tried to dry his eyes, but his tears kept coming.

The ED doctor started to get a bit irritated. There was nothing really wrong with Austin, and the doctor needed to see his next patient. Yet, he felt uncomfortable discharging a 15-year-old who was sobbing uncontrollably. What had the mother said? Austin had Asperger's? He asked if they felt that talking to a psychiatrist might help. Austin nodded yes again, and his head bobbed up and down rapidly.

"Call psych," the doctor told the nurse as he left Austin's room and hurried off. "Tell them the kid won't stop crying."

* * *

On busy nights, kids with a chief complaint of "crying" don't go to the head of the APS line. Just like on any other night, the psychiatry resident stuck covering the ED on New Year's Eve had to prioritize the patients who were suicidal or out of control. It would be hours before she would have time to see a crying teenager who had bruised his shoulder and couldn't seem to get over it.

The psychiatry resident answered the page from the nurse with the request for APS to see Austin.

"It will be a few hours," the resident said. "You sure they want to wait? And there's not much I can do for them now. Really, it would be better if they just went home, got some sleep, and came back the day after New Year's—preferably in the morning."

The nurse said she would check with Austin and his mother, but she was pretty sure that he, at least, wasn't going anywhere.

Sure enough, Austin waited and continued crying.

* * *

Around 4 A.M., Dr. N entered the room and saw Austin still sitting on the exam table. His eyes were red enough to match his hair, and he clutched crumpled tissues in his hand. His mother had left a few minutes before to get a cup of coffee and a snack at the all-night coffee shop in the main lobby of the hospital.

"Hi Austin, I'm Dr. N. I'm one of the psychiatrists in the ED tonight. I heard that you were feeling very sad."

"I suppose so. I keep crying," replied Austin, sniffling loudly.

"Why are you feeling sad?"

"I don't feel right. Nothing's right here. I hate it, I want to go home," said Austin.

"Where is home?" the resident asked.

"My mother and I came here last week. At my uncle's house, I had my room, and my books, and my telescope. I could watch the stars every night if I wanted to. I could see alpha Corona Borealis, you would know it as Gemma, beta Crucis, or Becrux, even Proxima Centauri . . . I could see them all from the porch." He twisted the tissues nervously in his hands, shredding them into little pieces, and started listing all of the stars that he knew.

"You must miss them," said Dr. N.

"I do," Austin agreed, tears streaming down his face. "I can't see anything here. I could barely even see Betelgeuse tonight! That's Alpha Orionis. My uncle says that city lights block out the stars."

"You know a lot about stars."

"I do. They're my friends," he said, and his shoulders started shaking as he tried to control his tears.

Dr. N sat down on one of the empty chairs and asked Austin more about his home, about what he missed, about what was important to him. Austin slowly told her about his mother's fight with his uncle, the bus ride, the shelter, and his worry that his uncle would just throw away his telescope. She learned that Austin had never seen a child psychiatrist. His pediatrician and his school counselor had helped him and his mother get the services he needed. She made sure that he wasn't so desperate that he felt like giving up and killing himself. His shoulder forgotten, the more Austin talked, the less he cried. He even started to smile a bit as he described his favorite astronomy book.

After a while, Dr. N said, "Austin, is Boston going to be your home now?"

"I think so. That's what my mom says anyway," he said somberly.

"Well, then we should wait until your mom gets back and think together about what we can do to make you feel more comfortable here. How does that sound?"

"Ok, I guess," he said.

* * *

Austin carried the diagnosis of Asperger's disorder, but that wasn't what brought him to the ED on New Year's Eve. He had also bumped his shoulder, but his bruise didn't require urgent attention. Austin came to the MGH on a cold night in Boston when everyone else seemed to have something to celebrate because he and his mother were in trouble, and they couldn't find anyone else to help.

The problems Austin and his mother faced fall into the category of socioeconomic disaster: the sudden move, the homeless shelter, financial hardship, uncertain future. The APS is frequently the final stop for children who suffer not from acute psychopathology but from social deprivation. Austin was certainly more vulnerable to becoming overwhelmed when faced with adverse circumstances than kids without Asperger's, but were it not for the chaos around him, he would probably not have shown up in the ED. Certainly, his complaints didn't require the skill set of a psychiatry resident: he didn't need a rapid diagnostic assessment; he didn't need medications; he didn't need to be hospitalized.

But he did need something. Austin, his mother, and Dr. N talked and planned for more than an hour that night. They talked about public observatories where Austin could go to see the stars, and after looking online, they located a dollar bookstore near his shelter where he might be able to find some more astronomy books. Dr. N told his mother how to have his Individualized Education Plan (IEP) transferred to his new school so that he could have a chance of getting into the small classroom he needed more quickly. She encouraged them to work with the social worker at the shelter, who had begun to help them access additional supports. They would need to apply for low-income housing and food stamps, find the appropriate plan within the state's health insurance system, and then arrange mental health services for Austin. Finally, she told Austin to call his uncle and ask him to put the telescope in a safe place until Austin and his mother could figure out a way to get it back.

When they were done talking, Dr. N wrote all of this information on Austin's discharge papers, making a list from the most important to the least important. She printed two copies of the discharge paper, one for Austin and one for his mother. It was now 6 A.M. Austin, no longer crying, headed back out into the cold with his mother and walked back toward the shelter.

Dr. N typed up her note in the emergency department's electronic medical record and wondered briefly if Austin and his mother would actually get the services she had described and what the uncle would do with Austin's precious telescope. Then she moved on.

* * *

New Year's Eve 2005. Another busy evening; the list of patients written on the white dry-erase board in the back room was getting longer. The residents were, as usual, busy seeing patients, typing their notes, or making calls. As luck would have it, Dr. N had pulled the same holiday coverage again.

The phone rang, and she picked it up.

"Is Dr. N there?" a young man's voice asked.

"Speaking. What can I do for you?" she answered.

"You probably won't remember me," he began. "I met you last year on New Year's Eve. My name is Austin."

At first Dr. N drew a blank, but something about the name rang a bell.

"Yes, I think I do," she said slowly, as a picture of a slightly chubby 15-year-old with red hair and freckles clutching tissues in his hands came to mind.

"I saw you exactly one year ago, and we talked," the boy on the phone continued. "You helped me feel better and I haven't forgotten. I kept the discharge paper you gave me, and it has this number on the bottom of it. I hope it's OK, but I just wanted to call and say thank you." He paused. "Oh, and my uncle didn't give away my telescope. I got it back."

"I am so glad to hear that," Dr. N said. "Thank you for calling. You really didn't have to."

"I wanted to," said Austin.

* * *

Austin still calls the APS every New Year's Eve. Dr. N does not work that holiday shift every year, but if she is not there, Austin always leaves a message for her with his thanks.

8

It's Just a Cold

Seventeen-year-old Elizabeth lay on a stretcher in a small examining room within the pediatrics section of the ED and stared at the TV suspended high in the corner of the room. She was tall and lean, with wispy blond hair that hung limp past her shoulders. Her mother, Mrs. T, sat in a chair next to her, still dressed in her business suit, several open file folders lying across her lap. She nervously twisted her necklace as she read the same paragraph over and over again, trying to keep her thoughts from returning to her daughter. Out of the corner of her eye, she watched her lying still on the stretcher, staring at the TV, captivated by it.

The TV was not on.

It didn't need to be. The overhead light created a reflection that seemed to bend and move across the screen. Elizabeth was certain that there was a message in that movement, but its meaning was hidden from her. She knew the message was critical; she just felt it. If she kept watching it, the meaning would be revealed to her.

Truth be told, Elizabeth hadn't really felt like herself since school started in September. She remembered last year, her junior year, how everything came so easily to her. Her classes were no problem; she got A's without even trying. She had tons of friends, and boys wanted to go out with her. But this year, something was different, off. She had nothing to say to her friends, so she got quieter and quieter, and then she just stopped talking to them altogether. She wasn't even interested in going out with boys anymore. It got so hard to pay attention in class, and the teachers seemed to be speaking faster and faster. When she tried to do her homework, her mind went blank. Her grades fell, which bummed her out at first. And then she just stopped caring altogether.

The curtain that separated the room from the hallway slid back and Dr. L, the ED pediatrician, entered. Mrs. T jumped to her feet and began talking immediately.

"Oh good—finally the doctor! My daughter's very sick—she has a terrible cold. She has fluid clogging up her whole head—it's so bad she can feel the fluid moving around. I described the symptoms to our pediatrician and he said to come right to the ED. I am sure he wanted us to get antibiotics," she explained.

Dr. L looked at Elizabeth and nodded, "All right. Elizabeth, I'm Dr. L. Tell me about this cold."

Elizabeth gazed at the doctor for a moment, smiling slightly, a small secret smile, as if she remembered a private joke she heard earlier in the day. "A few weeks ago, my head started to feel sort of funny. . . ." Her voice trailed off.

"Did you have a runny nose?" the doctor asked.

She shook her head no.

"A sore throat? A cough?"

She shook her head no again.

"A fever?"

"No."

"Headache?"

"No."

"OK, what did you have?"

After a long pause, Elizabeth said, "Well, there was the fluid, it kind of clogged up my head, and then my hearing got all weird."

"Weird how?" asked Dr. L.

Elizabeth shrugged her shoulders and looked away.

Dr. L did a physical examination. She rechecked Elizabeth's blood pressure and felt her wrist for her pulse. She listened to her heart and lungs, looked up her nostrils and in her throat and eyes, and spent a long time looking in her ears with the otoscope.

"Well, Elizabeth, your physical exam is normal. You look pretty healthy to me. And I don't see any fluid in your ear." Dr. L appeared slightly puzzled.

Elizabeth smiled oddly again and explained, with an air of certainty, "Oh, you can't see it, it's much deeper, and it's inside my brain, in the middle parts you can't see at all. It's a really special fluid though; it brings the perfect power with it. If I try really hard, I can make it move. I can feel it flowing through different parts of my brain. I can feel it right now. I keep trying to move it to the parts of my mind that do homework really well, but it mostly stays in the soccer playing parts. I guess that's all right though, we have an indoor tournament coming up."

It had been after she had stopped caring, after months of sleepwalking through each day, that she had begun to notice the fluid. She didn't know what it was at first; it started with just a small tickle in the middle of her brain. She kept noticing that tickle, and the more she noticed it, the stronger it grew. And then it started to move and flow, so she had realized the fluid was deep within her. At first, she was kind of worried that she might be sick or something, but then she noticed that the flowing fluid brought her a perfect power that gave her strength and confidence. Once again she could do some of the things she used to do—she was better at soccer (even if her coach didn't notice and left her on the bench all the time), and she could do her homework without a single mistake (even if the teacher said it was all wrong, she knew it was right). The puzzling part was that there wasn't quite enough fluid to cover her entire brain. She had to tilt her head to get the fluid to shift from one part to another.

As she thought these things, she tilted her head to the left and rested her ear on her shoulder. Then she slowly turned back to the TV.

Elizabeth's mom looked at the pediatrician, smiling nervously, "See what I mean, it's a very bad cold. Don't you get inner ear fluid, so deep you can't see it, with bad colds? Elizabeth keeps tilting her head so that the fluid will run out her ear. I am pretty sure she just needs those antibiotics and then we can be on our way. We've waited a long time already."

"Right, antibiotics," the pediatrician paused. "You know, I really need to speak with some other doctors about the best way to help Elizabeth. I am going to ask one of those doctors to come to talk with you. OK?" Without waiting for the answer, she spun around quickly and disappeared, pulling the curtain closed behind her.

Within minutes, Dr. L had paged the psychiatry resident.

"Hey, I need your help with a kid we have over in the Pedi side of the ED," she said. "She's a 17-year-old high school student who came in because she thinks she has a cold and maybe an ear infection. But her symptoms aren't from any cold I've ever seen. Something else is going on, something more in your area." Dr. L filled the psych resident in on the rest of the case.

"Does she really think that this fluid in her brain gives her special powers?"

"Seems like she does."

"Physical exam normal? Vital signs stable?"

"Yes. She's a healthy teen."

"Did you get a tox screen?"

"Oops. Will do."

"I'll see her after she's peed in a cup. Maybe this perfect power comes from some recreational drug."

"I don't think so," the pediatrician said, "but we'll check."

An hour later, Elizabeth's mom was still trying to read her files from work, when Dr. C, the psychiatry resident, entered the room.

Elizabeth's mom read the name tag and stood up, "Psychiatry? No, I don't think so. You are clearly in the wrong room. We are here because my daughter has a cold, a really bad one. It could be that Nile virus, no, I mean norovirus."

"I'm Dr. C," the resident said. "The pediatrician here asked me to come to see Elizabeth. We work together. I know that she will make sure Elizabeth gets the right treatment for her cold. Could I ask you to step out so that I could speak with Elizabeth privately for a few minutes?"

"No, whatever she has to say, she can say in front of her mother."

"Of course I want to hear what you think, also. But sometimes there are things that teenagers want to talk about without a parent present."

"Not in this case." Mrs. T was adamant.

Dr C looked at Elizabeth, who was still staring intently at the TV. "Elizabeth?" she asked.

Elizabeth looked back at her. She shrugged.

"Um, well . . . we'll at least get started. Elizabeth, Dr. L told me that you've been feeling some fluid in your brain. When did you first notice the fluid?"

"It was right around Thanksgiving, around when we went to New York," she said.

"I knew we shouldn't have gone there, you didn't get enough rest. It must have weakened your immune system," interrupted Elizabeth's mother.

"What else did you notice, Elizabeth?" asked Dr. C.

"Well," Elizabeth looked at her mom, not quite sure how to read her nervous stare, "the street signs were different, in New York I mean."

"Of course they were, honey, New York isn't Boston," her mom added.

"No, I mean, they were kind of giving me directions, like telling me the way I was supposed to go. It's hard to explain, but it was almost like they were pointing to the way I should walk."

"She went out with her older sister to go shopping and they got lost. I don't know why I ever let her go, it was terribly frightening," Elizabeth's mom filled in.

"Have you ever gotten other directions? Like a direction to hurt yourself or someone else? Have you ever felt that way?" asked Dr. C.

Elizabeth replied quickly, "No way. How could I hurt myself if I have the perfect power? That would just be crazy. And I have no reason to hurt anyone else. I don't even talk to other people."

"The perfect power?"

"Yeah, I told the other doctor. When the fluid in my brain flows to one part, that part works the best.

"OK, Elizabeth. What else have you noticed?" asked Dr. C.

"That other doctor asked about my hearing, it got all weird."

"Isn't that a sign of an ear infection?" Elizabeth's mother interjected.

"It could be," replied Dr. C. "Go on, Elizabeth."

"It wasn't that my hearing got worse, like that doctor said. It was more like I could hear extra stuff, like a gift, you know?" She said, looking at Dr. C, who nodded. "The thoughts other people were thinking, I could hear them all the time."

"Could you hear voices? Voices that other people couldn't hear?" asked Dr. C.

Elizabeth's mom interrupted again. "Now wait, what kind of question is that? My daughter isn't hearing voices. How dare you imply that! My daughter has a bad cold. We came here to get antibiotics. We don't need a psychiatrist, and you are clearly confusing her with all of your questions. She's saying things she doesn't really mean. You need to leave now."

"Mrs. T, I'm worried about Elizabeth," said Dr. C.

"Well, you don't need to, she will be just fine. This is a temporary problem. My daughter has never, ever had psychiatric problems. Leave now; your time with my daughter is over. I won't permit you to speak with her any further," Mrs. T said forcefully.

Dr. C started to open her mouth again.

"No," said Mrs. T firmly, "you will not ask one more question of my daughter. You have done enough damage already. You are done here, doctor. Done." She sat back down in her chair and picked up her papers. "Ask the other doctor to come back in here and we will talk about what medication Elizabeth needs."

"Mrs. T, I understand you are upset. Please let me take a few minutes to speak with the child psychiatry fellow on call. I'll be back in a few minutes."

* * *

As soon as the doctor left the room, Mrs. T turned to her daughter and whispered, "Get your clothes on now, we are leaving this place. This is a mad house."

Elizabeth took her clothes out of the green plastic hospital bags she had put them in when she first arrived. She dressed quickly, not quite understanding, but following her mother's directions. When she was dressed, Mrs. T stuck her head out from behind the curtain and scanned both sides of the hallway. It was empty.

"Come on now, let's go," she whispered again.

The two walked quickly out of the room and down the hall toward the door marked "Exit." On the other side, they found themselves in a wide corridor.

"Do you remember which way to go?" she asked her daughter.

Elizabeth looked at the signs on the wall and smiled that secret smile again, "I don't remember exactly, but I can figure it out."

She tilted her head to her shoulder, closed her eyes for a moment, and then pointed to the left. The two walked past stretchers full of patients lining the hallways, around the corner, through the waiting room, into a larger lobby, down a much wider corridor, and out the front door of the hospital. The cool night air hit them as they exited. Mrs. T kept her head low, her eyes down to the ground, saying over and over, "It's just a cold, just a cold." Elizabeth stopped before they entered the garage to find their car. She looked up at the midnight sky as if reading signs in the stars that were visible only to her.

* * * * *

"Where did they go?" Dr. C asked the nurse assigned to Elizabeth's room.
"Who?"
"Elizabeth and her mother?"
"They're in room 3."
"Not any more."
"What do you mean?"
"No one's there now. Room's empty."
"You're kidding." The nurse rushed down the corridor to see for herself. She walked slowly back. "Gone, gone, gone. Do you think I have to send security to look for them?"

Dr. C thought a minute. "No. We can try calling the mother's cell phone number, if she left it with us, although I'm pretty sure she won't answer it."

"Well, we've got to do something. She wasn't discharged yet."

"I'll check with my attending, but I can't send the paramedics to her door and bring her back here against her will just because she thinks there's a fluid in her brain that moves around and confers special powers. She's not dangerous to herself or to anyone else. She goes to school. What did her tox screen show?" she asked as an afterthought.

"It was negative. No drugs. So, what did you think was wrong with her?"

"I think she is having a first psychotic break."

"Really?"

"She's having hallucinations, losing touch with reality. Her concentration's off, she's too distracted by her thoughts to remember things. She believes that the street signs are giving her personal messages. She's not depressed, so I don't think this is related to her mood. Don't know. Might be the first sign of schizophrenia; might not."

"Isn't there anything else we should do? She seemed like a nice kid."

"Well, we can at least call the pediatrician who referred her to us and let that doc know what we think. Maybe he can help us negotiate with the mother. The kid needs a workup, that's for sure. Short of that, we'll just have to wait."

* * *

Kids who are experiencing their first break with reality can be both frightened and frightening. Some are terrified by their thoughts, convinced that others intend to hurt them, even family members or other loved ones. Elizabeth's situation was a bit different. She felt puzzled by what was happening, but she was not upset. Her delusion—her idea that the fluid in her head carried a perfect power that could lead her to the right answer—was actually reassuring to her. But her mother was not reassured. Indignant protests notwithstanding, at some level, she probably recognized that the fluid in her daughter's head was not due to an upper respiratory tract infection and that her daughter's conviction that the street signs in New York were pointing out the proper route was not due to lack of sleep.

The ED is often the place where both patients and family members first confront the idea that their signs and symptoms are part of a larger, more complex and truly worrisome picture. When the psychiatry resident started asking Elizabeth if she had ever heard voices outside her head, Elizabeth's mother began to realize that the doctors thought her daughter had a mental health problem, not an infection. Mother panicked and fled the ED with Elizabeth, hoping, perhaps, that in leaving the questions unanswered, she was also leaving the problems behind.

If her mother's history is correct, Elizabeth had never had any contact with a mental health professional before. Her symptoms had not come on acutely, but they were, nevertheless, of fairly recent onset. A first psychotic episode like this can be triggered by severe mood symptoms similar to those one might see in depression or mania; it can be a reaction to severe trauma, medications, or illicit drugs; it can be due to a primary psychotic disorder, such as schizophrenia—a complex disorder in which the exact biological cause of the symptoms is, as yet, unknown.

Sometimes, the kind of delusions that Elizabeth experienced can accompany underlying medical problems such as seizure disorders, brain tumors, occult central nervous system infections, or metabolic abnormalities. Even though Elizabeth had had a physical exam in the ED, such exams are, by their nature, symptom-focused with the goal of ruling out any life-threatening problem; a more in-depth examination may be deferred to the outpatient department.

Elizabeth's negative urine screen for toxins like amphetamines, cannabinoids, barbiturates, opiates, or other drugs made it unlikely that medication or recreational drug use was the cause of her problem. The absence of a history of mood symptoms of any kind, severe depression, or euphoria also suggested that the cause of her symptoms lay elsewhere.

But, given the large number of potential causes for her presentation, Elizabeth needed a more extensive workup, including laboratory tests to evaluate the functioning of her liver, kidneys, and thyroid, as well as tests to make sure she did not have an infection or autoimmune disease. She would also need imaging studies of her head like a computerized tomography (CT) scan or magnetic resonance imaging (MRI) to rule out any intracranial cause of mental status change, such as a brain tumor, and potentially an electroencephalogram (EEG) to make sure she was not having seizures.

* * *

Dr. C paged Elizabeth's pediatrician in the middle of the night to explain what had happened. "Do you think you could call the mom in the morning? Any chance you could reason with her and get her to bring the kid back? It's not the usual way things work, but if it would make a difference, I would be willing to see them in the outpatient clinic; maybe that would be less scary."

The pediatrician promised to try.

The next morning, the pediatrician called Mrs. T at home. He acknowledged how worried the doctors were and emphasized the seriousness of the situation. Somewhat reluctantly, Mrs. T agreed to bring Elizabeth back to the outpatient clinic but not to the emergency room to finish answering the doctor's questions and to complete the workup her daughter needed. She and Elizabeth were on time for their appointment. After a more lengthy discussion with Dr. C and her supervisor in the outpatient clinic, both Elizabeth and her mother agreed to the tests the doctors thought were necessary.

Ultimately, Dr. C diagnosed Elizabeth with schizophrenia and began to treat her with a combination of medication and supportive therapy. Elizabeth did very well; after a period of some months, she was able to return to high school. She graduated a year late but maintained a few friendships and eventually headed off to college.

9

CHILDREN COME WITH PARENTS

One Sunday afternoon, six-year-old Franklin was late for drop-off at his dad's house. He was supposed to be back at his dad's house by 5:00 P.M. on Sunday. But tonight, at exactly 5:00 P.M., he was sitting in the triage area of the ED, while his mother explained to the psychiatry resident, Dr. M, why she had brought her son to the MGH. Franklin was small for his age, a scrawny kid; his knobby knees were visible below his oversized shorts. He sat very still and watched his mother with solemn brown eyes.

"Franklin's not himself, he's out of control, something's very wrong. I know he's supposed to be at his father's by 5 P.M. today, but I just couldn't send him back there knowing something was so wrong with him. Please help me. You do understand, don't you?" Mrs. R said, her pleading words tumbling out quickly.

Earlier today, she and Franklin had been at the Aquarium. Franklin had seen all of the exhibits and raced up and down the ramp that spiraled around the huge fish tank for at least an hour. At the end of the day, shortly before his mother had to drive Franklin to his father's house, they went to the gift shop. His mother planned to buy him a toy to take with him to his father's. But Franklin wasn't ready to leave. He wanted to see one more turtle, a special turtle, before they left. As he and his mother approached the gift shop, Franklin began to yell at her, kick his feet, and clench his fists. His mother tried to gather him in her arms and give him a hug, but he wouldn't let her near him. When she reached for him, he hit her and then he shoved her. She had cried out, attracting a bit of attention from other Aquarium-goers. When someone asked her if she needed help, she said no, and dragged Franklin, who was now crying, out of the Aquarium and back to her car.

"I've never seen him like this—so angry, so inconsolable. I don't understand what set him off; we had a wonderful day." Then, she added, "I left a message on his dad's cell phone, so he should know we're here." She rubbed her arm where Franklin had hit her.

Mrs. R explained that, since the divorce was finalized, Franklin spent alternating weeks with each parent.

"Who has legal custody of Franklin?" Dr. M asked.

This is one of the first and most important questions in any emergency child psychiatric evaluation. We cannot evaluate or treat a minor child without the consent of the custodial figure. Certainly, we cannot discharge a child to the care of someone who is not legally responsible for him or her. If a child lives with both parents, we usually assume that both parents share custody. If they are separated, divorced, never married, or remarried to another person, then we always ask. Determining who has custody can be difficult. A stepparent may be the primary caregiver, but if he or she has not adopted the child, then he or she has no custodial rights. If DCF has assumed custody in cases where the parents are unfit, a representative from that agency must come to the APS to be with the child. Custody can also be split. For example, one parent can hold physical custody (where the child resides) and both parents can share legal or decision-making custody, or the court can appoint a relative to hold physical custody and DCF can retain legal custody.

Mrs. R reported that, according to the divorce agreement, she and her husband shared legal custody, which meant that either parent could consent to an emergency medical evaluation or a hospitalization, even without the presence or agreement of the other. It also meant that both parents had equal say in what happened to their child. If they were both present in the ED and they disagreed about whether to follow the psychiatrist's recommendations, then things could get ugly.

"Where is your ex-husband now?" Dr. M asked.

"He'll show up, I guarantee you," she said, "Right, Franklin?"

With that, Mrs. R and Franklin walked quietly with Dr. M toward the APS. Whatever had caused Franklin's tantrum, it had been short-lived.

* * *

A young child, like Franklin, will usually be able to tell a story about why he is in the ED but not be able to place his story in context. For this reason, residents almost always choose to talk with the parent or guardian first in order to obtain the background information that will inform their interview of the child.

The APS was not busy. A nurse directed Franklin to one of the interview rooms and Mrs. R to another one. She offered each one some ginger ale and crackers. Franklin shyly nodded yes to the question about a snack. Mrs. R, a thin woman who looked haggard and defeated, said no.

Dr. M chose to start with Franklin's mother.

Mrs. R twisted a tight, bleached blonde curl around her finger as she launched in to her story: Franklin had had tantrums at drop-off before, but not like this. She was sure that he hated going to his father's house and that he was unhappy when he was there. His father made Franklin feel bad about himself all the time. That's why Franklin had lost it. She was positive. Someone needed to get to the bottom of this right away. It was no accident that this had happened when she was supposed to bring Franklin back to his father. Her son needed to be evaluated. Now. She would never, ever put that court-ordered transfer above her son's well-being.

"So you think that Franklin hit you because he didn't want to go to his father's house?"

"He's been having these tantrums more and more, but I finally realized that they are the worst just before I have to take him over to his dad's. I don't know why he has to go back and forth like this. It's not good for him. His father is a very angry man."

* * *

One of the nurses knocked on the door and poked her head in the interview room, "I do believe that the child's father has arrived," she told Dr. M.

"Give me another minute or two and I'll be right there," Dr. M said.

She turned back to Mrs. R. "Did your husband hit you? Are you worried that he will hurt Franklin?"

"I don't know what happens over there."

"But did he used to hit you?"

"He can be very threatening," she insisted.

"Did he ever hurt you?"

"No."

"Or Franklin?"

"I don't think so," she admitted.

"Can you please wait with Franklin?" She asked Mrs. R. "He's right next door."

* * *

Franklin's father was a compact, powerful-looking man, only about 5 feet 8 inches tall, but with a broad, dense body. His thick neck spilled over the collar of his shirt, and several small healing cuts were just visible. He waited in triage. As Dr. M approached, he stood up.

She introduced herself and extended her hand. He ignored her greeting.

"What is going on with my son?" He raised his voice. "What did that crazy bitch do now? She left me a message that she brought him here."

Dr. M explained that Franklin was having some ginger ale and crackers and that his mother had brought him because he had become out of control when the two of them were visiting the Aquarium.

Irritated, he said, "Look lady, I know my kid. There's nothing wrong with him, nothing that stupid mother of his hasn't created in her own sick mind. She sees crazy everywhere, but the crazy's just in her. She says he's 'maladjusted,' so now I've got to bring him to a therapist every week, and pay for it, too. She keeps telling people he's sick, but I'll tell you, my kid's normal. He's a happy, 'adjusted' kid when he's with me. She's the crazy one. She did this the last time she dropped him off," he said, pointing to the scratches on his neck, "when I wouldn't let her inside to keep saying goodbye!" His fists were clenched and his voice got louder and louder. "You know, I'd really like to just take my son out of here. But I don't want to give her any ammunition to use against me in court. She hates it that Franklin spends time at my house. So, go ahead, talk to him. See for yourself there's nothing wrong. Call his therapist, he sees him every week. But be quick, I want to take my son home. This is my time with Franklin." He stared hard at the doctor.

Dr. M looked around. People were milling about, but no one was paying much attention to the conversation between the two of them. He made her nervous. She wished she had thought to ask the security guards to accompany her to triage to meet the father.

She backed up slightly. "Mr. R," she said, "I understand that you're upset and that you think Franklin is fine. But once someone brings a child to this ED, we have to evaluate him. His mother believes that the child is afraid to go to your home. I will have to ask you to wait while we sort this out." With that, she turned quickly and headed back into the relative safety of the APS.

* * *

Dr. M returned to the interview room and found Franklin sitting on his mother's lap, his head on her shoulder. As she entered, he looked up quickly.

"Hey Franklin, would it be OK if you and I spent some time together? We could draw or play or do anything you like."

Franklin looked at his mother and saw the tears in her eyes. "I want to stay with my mom. Mom, I want to be with you." And he leaned over to hug her, keeping his eyes on the doctor.

"Your mom can stay right here and we'll go next door. If you want her while we're talking, we'll come get her. Let's give it a try. It's important."

He looked at his mom. "Is it okay?" She nodded yes. He looked at her for a moment longer, making sure she was not going to change her mind. She nodded again, and he hopped off the chair and followed Dr. M out the door and into the other interview room.

Dr. M opened up one of the drawers and took out markers and paper. She placed them on the desk and asked him if he wanted to draw.

"I don't feel like drawing," he said.

"Do you know why you are here today?" she asked gently.

"Yes," said Franklin, solemnly. "I was at the Aquarium, and I got very mad, and now I am in trouble."

"Franklin, you aren't in trouble. We're just here to talk. Can you tell me what happened at the Aquarium today?" asked Dr. M.

Franklin nodded his head vigorously; he seemed relieved that he was not in trouble. He explained that after they saw all those interesting sea creatures, they headed to the gift shop so that he could choose a toy to bring to his dad's. His mom kept telling him to hurry up; she said they couldn't be late for his dad's house because of what happened last time. But he wanted to see the big turtle once more. She kept saying hurry, hurry, and he remembered how angry his mom and dad were at the last drop-off, how they were yelling, and fighting. . . . His voice began to trail off.

"You must have been very, very mad to hit her," said Dr. M.

He looked away from her but nodded his head.

"Do you feel mad often?" asked Dr. M.

He shook his head no. "Not that often."

"What makes you mad?" asked Dr. M.

He thought for a few moments. "When I can't have an ice cream after dinner. Or when I have to clean up my toys."

"Anything else?"

"Nope. But it's really hard to clean up my toys. I have a lot," he paused. "More at my dad's house."

Dr. M pressed on, "How about scared? Do you get scared?"

"Sometimes."

"Like when?" she asked.

"When it rains, if there's lightning and thunder. That's scary. Or if my room's too dark, that's scary too. Or when I have a bad dream. Once I had a dream about a clown that was very scary."

"Do grown-ups ever scare you?"

"Uh huh. There's an old man who lives next to my dad, and he's got a big dog he walks on a leash, and sometimes the dog barks, and I'm scared the old man will let him go and he will run at me."

"Tell me about your dad's house."

"I have my own room, with a race car bed. And I have a play room, with lots of toys. And I have books, too. I like books."

"Is it ever scary at Dad's house?"

He looked up at her as if he didn't understand the questions.

"I mean aside from when it's dark, or when there is thunder. Is it ever scary other times?" she continued.

He looked puzzled. "No, it's not scary. My dad is there. He's strong."

"I see. What's the best part of being at your dad's?"

"We play Cookie Man. Do you know that game? It's really fun. We play that our house is a cookie store, and we can make any cookies we want. My dad has special cookie dough, and he puts the cookies on the baking sheet. Then I choose what to put on top, I can choose anything I want. I like to put on sprinkles, or a Hershey's kiss, or sometimes raisins. And I get to put them on, all by myself. And then we bake the cookies and we get to eat them!"

"Well, just one at a time," he added as an afterthought.

"That sounds like fun. What is the worst part of being at your dad's?"

"I have to take a bath every day."

"A bath every day? That is hard!"

He giggled a bit.

"How about your mom's house? What is the best part of being at your mom's?"

"She reads me stories every night at bedtime. We snuggle in bed, and she reads me as many stories as I want."

"That sounds nice. What's the worst part?"

He paused for a moment and stared down at his lap. "When I have to leave. She always gets sad and hugs me a lot. And then my dad gets mad because it takes too long. And then they fight. They fight a lot. They told me that when they didn't live together they would stop fighting," he said.

"I see. You worry that your mother will be sad because you go away to your dad's. But you really like to be at your dad's."

He nodded vigorously.

"And when your mom gets sad, your dad gets mad, and then they argue."

He whispered a small "Yes."

"And when they argue, you feel sad too. . . . And mad."

He nodded and then hiccupped.

"What happens when your dad gets angry?"

"He yells. He yells a lot. He yells at my mom."

"Has he ever hurt you?"

"No."

"You sure?"

Franklin nodded.

"I bet you just want to skip the drop-off."

"I hate drop-off," he said.

"I see. I think I understand better now. You did a good job of explaining this to me."

"Did my dad come?"

"Yes, he's here."

"Good. I'm supposed to be with him now."

Franklin smiled a small smile, and he looked at the markers. Dr. M pushed them over to him. "You can draw if you wanted to. I need to make some phone calls, but you can stay here and draw. I would love to see a picture of your family—could you draw me a picture of your family?" He smiled again and picked up a blue marker.

* * *

A phone call to Franklin's therapist, who had been seeing him every week for more than a year, confirmed that Franklin's tantrums were most often triggered by his anticipating or witnessing conflict between his parents. The therapist was not worried that the child was developing a major mental illness but was very concerned about how the persistent acrimony was affecting him. Usually, Franklin was talkative and active, with lots of interests; he wasn't depressed or withdrawn. He loved school and had many friends. He was clearly attached to each parent. The therapist had tried to talk with both mother and father about their behavior, but they refused to stay in the same room together long enough to make any meaningful joint decisions. He had concluded that the parents couldn't stand the idea that they had to share their son's attention: "I bet they're on the phone to their lawyers all the time, plotting how to get the custody arrangement changed."

"Do you think Franklin is in any danger at either parent's house?" Dr. M asked him. "Mrs. R feels that Franklin gets so upset because he is anxious about spending a week with his father."

"Danger?" he repeated. "No. I don't believe he's ever been in danger. Both his mother and his father hate it when Franklin likes something about the other parent. Mother buys Franklin a toy before she lets him go to his father's house, as if to imply that the father won't give him enough. And father always refers to his ex-wife as 'that bitch' or 'that crazy bitch' or even worse. The irony is that Franklin really loves both his parents."

* * *

Dr. M asked one of the security guards to join her while she spoke with Franklin's parents. She then ushered the parents into a separate office, away from where Franklin was drawing. No one sat down. The former husband and wife stared at each other with contempt. Dr. M leaned her back against the wall. The security guard lounged just outside the doorway.

For a moment, no one spoke.

Mr. R began, "I can't believe you have pulled this crap, you stupid bitch. You are the one screwing up this kid, not me."

Mrs. R shot back, "At least I care for our son; at least I am looking out for his well-being. You couldn't care less, you selfish pig."

Dr. M interrupted and asked, "Are you here to fight with one another or are you here because of Franklin?"

"We wouldn't be here at all if she," the father pointed at his ex-wife, "wasn't sure that Franklin hated me as much as she does."

"What did you find? What did he tell you? He's in crisis, isn't he?" Mrs. R said quickly.

The father slammed his hand down on the desk, "Franklin is not in crisis."

"So what is wrong with my son?" the mother asked defensively.

Mr. R said through pursed lips, "There's nothing wrong with my son."

Dr. M interrupted them again. "The two of you need to stop arguing if you want to leave here tonight. You have a lovely child. Franklin can't handle the fighting. Something here has got to give."

"Well, what plan do you suggest, doctor?" asked Mr. R sarcastically. "Try to tell this woman anything. Go ahead."

"At the very least, it is critical that you have a different plan for your son's drop-off. You cannot continue to do this to Franklin. He doesn't have a psychiatric diagnosis right now, but if this continues, he will certainly be at risk for one. It's not my job to tell you how to feel or even how to treat one another. What you do in private is your business. But it is my job to make sure that Franklin is safe. For right now, you need a third party to do this drop-off so you two won't be in contact with each other in front of him, at least until you can figure out a way to get along. Call your lawyers if you must, but no one goes home until you make a plan. No one."

Dr. M said all of this with an air of conviction that belied the fact that she knew she had no right to insist on any of it.

Truth be told, she had already determined that Franklin was not in any acute danger. There were none of the so-called safety issues to worry about. Mother believed that father was frightening their son, but Franklin didn't seem frightened. In fact, he liked being with his father. He didn't need to be admitted to an inpatient unit or medicated. There was no need to alert DCF, as mother was not alleging actual abuse or neglect. Even the outpatient therapist felt that Franklin was safe with either parent. The custody arrangement specified that Franklin was to be dropped off at 5 P.M. at his father's. Mother was in violation of that order. Father had every right to take the child home with him. Mother couldn't stop him and neither could Dr. M.

* * *

Down the hall, Franklin had finished his picture. "I finished the picture for you, see?" he said excitedly, holding the paper out to the doctor.

"Yes, that's great. What did you draw?"

He pointed at the drawing, "This me, and this is my mom and this is my dad. It's my whole family. I don't have any brothers or sisters yet."

Franklin had drawn himself in the center of the page, standing tall, with stick arms and legs, and a straight mouth, no smile. To his left was his mother, also a stick figure; she had yellow curls and one of her arms extended out toward the child in the middle, almost touching him. On his other side, Franklin had drawn his father. Also a stick figure, the lines of his body were thicker and his hair was black. He, too, had an arm held out to the child.

* * *

One of the security guards walked Mrs. R back to one of the interview rooms, and another security guard took Mr. R to the other one. With the assistance of their respective lawyers, they did work out a different plan for Sunday evenings. The father's parents agreed to bring the child from one house to another. Mother, at the urging of her attorney, agreed to this plan.

Dr. M brought Franklin to say goodbye to his mother. He hugged her. Then she brought Franklin to his father. Mr. R lifted him up and carried him out of the APS. It was 9 P.M.

* * *

This is a simple story with a seemingly predictable ending. Franklin is certainly not the only six-year-old ever to have had a tantrum at the end of a long day at the Aquarium. Yet, he had to spend four hours in a major metropolitan hospital's emergency room—all because one of his parents could not bear to relinquish him to the other, not even when under strict court order to do so.

When the APS becomes yet another battlefield for parents locked in combat, it can be difficult for the staff to stay out of the fray. Did Dr. M overstep her bounds? She saw her role as advocate for Franklin; she voiced his frustration, pain, anger, and sadness. Can we understand her ultimatum to the parents as another version of the father's bullying and the mother's scratching and the child's pushing and shoving? She, too, met fire with fire.

In this case, Dr. M was fortunate. The parents backed down and allowed her to dictate their actions. But the case could have gone another way. Father could have simply left with Franklin. Mother could have become increasingly argumentative, upped the ante, and accused the father of abuse or neglect, forcing a call to DCF and a delay in discharge. Did Dr. M make a difference in the life of this child? In the short term, yes. In the long term, who knows?

10

Little Bear

"I . . . want . . . a . . . bear!" Dahlia's high-pitched scream filled the ED. "I WANT A BEAR!! I WANT A BEAR!!"

Patients lying on stretchers in the hallway groaned. The maintenance worker in a blue polo shirt pushing an empty trash can down the corridor stopped and turned his head toward the sound.

A hospital volunteer practically flew down the hallway carrying a small stuffed brown bear with a red ribbon at its neck in one hand.

"I found one!" she cried before disappearing through the door that led to the pediatric section of the ED and into a patient room.

A moment of silence was followed by a crash and a yell.

"I . . . don't . . . want . . . this . . . bear!!!!!" the same high-pitched voice began again, "I . . . want . . . a . . . different . . . one!!!!!!"

* * *

Marie, Dahlia's biological mother, had struggled with depression and drug abuse for much of her life. During her pregnancy with Dahlia, she continued to shoot heroin and cocaine. At birth, Dahlia weighed four pounds and was addicted to opiates. After several weeks in the hospital, she went home with Marie under the watchful eye of DCF. But being a new mother was too tough; Marie quickly slipped back into a life of intravenous drug use. Six months later, the DCF took Dahlia away from her mother and placed her in foster care. After a court hearing, Marie's parental rights were terminated. She never saw Dahlia again.

By her third birthday, Dahlia had lived with three different foster families. The third placement was at the home of a middle-aged couple who had no children of their own. They adored Dahlia and decided to adopt her. She was a bit hyperactive, but her new parents could keep up with her. She had trouble sleeping, but they could tag-team her. She sometimes bit her own arm, and once she had even bitten the arm of a younger child who was visiting the home. Her parents accessed services through the state and placed Dahlia in a specialized preschool where the teachers could help her with her behavior.

Shortly after her fourth birthday, Dahlia started to have explosive tantrums that occurred several times each day and lasted for hours at a time. Her parents did everything the parenting books said to do—ignored the tantrums, praised calm behavior, created a safe time-out space. But the tantrums got worse; Dahlia threw dishes, broke toys and gadgets, banged her head against the wall, and tried to hit her parents. Sometimes plopping her down in front of a television set was the only thing they could do to calm her.

Almost all preschoolers have temper tantrums. As they try to gain mastery over small tasks by doing them independently, they often become frustrated and irritable when they can't do what they want to do. Frustration can quickly turn into a tantrum, especially because younger children aren't always able to express their feelings in words. But few toddlers or preschoolers have tantrums like Dahlia's.

Dahlia's pediatrician recommended that her parents take her to see a psychologist, who diagnosed her with attention deficit hyperactivity disorder, intermittent explosive disorder, and a mood disorder. She started weekly play therapy, but her tantrums continued. The psychologist sent her to a neurologist and then a developmental pediatrician. They worried about genetic/metabolic disorders or structural brain changes, yet all of her imaging studies, chromosomal analysis, and other blood tests were normal.

Finally, someone referred the family to a child psychiatrist in the community. The psychiatrist diagnosed juvenile bipolar disorder and recommended medication, but the parents were reluctant as they were aware of the risks and uncertain about the benefits. For a while, they preferred to manage her with behavioral management strategies and hope.

Then one day, Dahlia almost tore the ear off Lucky, the family's puppy. Even their vet didn't believe that a little girl could do something like that. That was it. The parents went back to see the child psychiatrist and asked for some medication for Dahlia.

The atypical neuroleptic the doctor chose helped a little bit. Now Dahlia could sometimes sleep through the night; she was a little bit less impulsive during the day but still unpredictable and volatile. One particularly bad day, however, Dahlia grew out of control when playing tag with kids in the neighborhood. She grabbed another girl's arm and wouldn't let go. While the other girl struggled, Dahlia continued to pull on her arm as if she were playing tug-of-war. The other girl ended up in a local ED with a dislocated shoulder. Dahlia ended up in the APS; from there she was transferred to a psychiatric unit for the first time. She was four years old.

The cycle began. Dahlia would spend a few weeks on an inpatient unit where the doctors would add or subtract medications, the social worker would review the in-home behavior plans, and the parents would get some rest. Then, she would be discharged to her parents with in-home services.

In an effort to keep children out of the hospital, the state has poured resources into community-based programs that provide services like in-home therapy (a therapist who goes to the home to work with kids and families), intensive care coordination (an intensive case manager), and therapeutic mentorship (a therapeutic "big brother/sister"). The goal is to offer children and their families enough support in the community to prevent hospitalization. Dahlia's family qualified for such services and accepted them gladly.

Dahlia would do well at home for a brief time before, despite the best intentions of her in-home team, her aggressive and out-of-control behavior would resume, and her parents would call the outpatient psychiatrist. Before long, Dahlia would end up back in the ED.

* * *

An APS nurse walked into the back work room where the residents, attending, and nurse-practitioner were busy typing notes and answering the constantly ringing phone. She announced, "Just got a call from triage, Dahlia's back. She's out of control as usual, headed to pediatrics as we speak."

One resident sighed loudly, just as another said, "Again? How can that be? She was just here."

Dr. G, the attending psychiatrist, said, "Well, she's here," then asked, "Who's willing to see her?"

"I had her last time," one said as he turned back to his computer and resumed typing.

"And I had her the time before that," the other one muttered. "Isn't there something we can do about these little repeat offenders? I mean, the adults who drop in to see us every week get case managers and hospital diversion plans."

"This is a four-year-old," Dr. G pointed out. "Four-year-olds don't get hospital diversion plans. They shouldn't have to be in psych hospitals to begin with."

"Well this little four-year-old needs something," the resident persisted. "But I don't think it's me," he laughed.

"You guys are too new at this to be burnt out," Dr. G shot back.

"Dahlia's one of those kids from Krypton," the same resident persisted. "Leaping tall buildings in a single bound. Watch out."

"Never mind, I'll see her myself," Dr. G said.

Hospitalizing a child of any age is a big deal, but hospitalizing a four-year-old is an even bigger deal. Referring a child to an inpatient psychiatric unit means separating her from her parents and taking her away from all that is familiar—house, bed, toys, friends—and exposing her to other, often older kids with mental health problems. Few units allow parents to stay with their children overnight.

For little kids, hospitalization is thus an intervention reserved for the most extreme situations. The goal is to protect the child and those around him or her, when no other means can maintain safety. Hospitalization also allows for rapid medication changes and intensive family therapy to bring things quickly under control. It can offer respite to parents who are usually beyond exhausted from caring for such a severely ill child.

* * *

Dr. G walked over to the pediatric side of the ED and peeked through the small window set in the door of the examining room. She saw Dahlia, now calmer, sitting on her father's lap, and focused on the TV set in the corner of the room. Dahlia's mother caught her eye and came out of the room. Dr. G nodded hello, and the two found a quiet place to sit in an adjacent empty examining room.

"So tell me what's happened since the last time Dahlia was here?" Dr. G asked. "I don't think we've met before, but I certainly have heard about Dahlia."

"Everyone knows Dahlia," mother sighed. "I feel like we live here. She just got out of the hospital a week and a half ago. She started on a new medication, and got a new in-home therapist. I was feeling good about it," she added.

"What went wrong?"

Mother continued, "She did better for a few days, and then it all started up again. She hasn't been sleeping much, just four or five hours a night, and when she's awake, she keeps getting into things—she smeared playdough all over the walls of her room, and she even pushed over a small table. My husband and I took shifts sleeping so someone could watch her at all times. I tried to hold out over the weekend because I knew we had a doctor's appointment today at the clinic. I thought we could make it. I really wanted to make it."

"And then what happened today?" asks Dr. G.

"At first, Dahlia was excited to be there in the outpatient clinic, but then a switch just flipped. We were still in the waiting room and she started screaming when she had to take a turn on the chalkboard with another child. And then she just wouldn't stop. She crawled under the chairs, and I couldn't coax her out. She just lay there yelling. The secretary called our doctor to come out, and when the doctor came out to see us, Dahlia ran past him, right into the office. She seemed calmer for a few minutes, but then she went off again. She started yelling and stomping her feet. Even the doctor couldn't quiet her down. Then she started throwing things; she was just grabbing everything within her reach and throwing it. She hit the doctor in the head with a stapler he had on his desk. That may have been what did it. It's amazing that her dad was able to carry her down here to the ED."

"Oh, I see," said Dr. G, wondering if the outpatient doc was getting stitches in some other part of the ED. "Do you think there's something in particular that sets her off?"

Mother replied, "You can never tell what's going to set her off. It could be anything. Sure, she gets upset at the normal things—being told that it's bedtime, having to pick up her toys, not getting to have an extra cookie—but she also gets upset for no reason. She can be having a wonderful time playing outside, or reading a story, and then she just suddenly loses it. Lately, she has been getting even more aggressive."

"Hard to imagine her being much worse," said Dr. G.

"She's been kicking, hitting, biting, throwing things. . . . She did this." The mother pulled up her sleeve; her arm was covered in bruises from her wrist up past her elbow. "When I try to hold her, she often bites my arm, right through my shirt."

Dr. G didn't say anything.

Mother looked at Dr. G's face and then looked away. She continued, "But Dahlia isn't a bad kid; she feels terrible afterwards. She knows she's doing something wrong, but once she gets going, she can't stop."

* * *

The two walked together back into the pediatric examining room. Dahlia was still sitting on her father's lap. Her eyes were on the TV, but her body was in constant motion. Her legs swung back and forth, banging into her father's shins. Her hands tapped a rhythm against her thighs, her fists clenched and opened, her body rocked forward and back, kept in check only by her father's arms wrapped around her torso.

Dr. G bent down to her eye level and said, "Hey Dahlia, I'm Dr. G. I've actually heard quite a bit about you. Do you know why you are here today?"

She turned her round blue eyes away from the TV and looked at the doctor. "No," she said.

"Dahlia, your mom and dad and doctor are worried about how upset you got today. Did you know that?"

"No, I'm watching TV. Did you see "Finding Nemo"?" asked Dahlia.

"I did see "Finding Nemo." I liked it, too," said Dr. G. "What's your favorite part?"

"I like it when Marlin and Dory ride the current with the turtles—they go fast! I like going fast!" said Dahlia.

"I liked that part, too," said Dr. G.

"And the part where Nemo goes down the drain? That was good too. And the part with the jellyfish, I liked that part too. I like Nemo," Dahlia talked rapidly, keeping her eyes glued to the screen.

"Maybe we can talk for a few minutes and then you can watch the rest of Nemo. Let's turn this off for just a minute," suggested Dr. G.

That was a mistake.

As soon as Dr. G turned the TV off, Dahlia tried to squirm out of her father's grip.

Father looked to Dr. G for a direction.

"You can let her down if you like," she said.

Father let go, and Dahlia jumped off his lap. She dashed around the room, pulled boxes off the metal supply shelves that lined the back wall, and threw them into the air. Her parents called her name, trying to get her attention. No go. Soon she began to yell "No, no, no" over and over again, at top volume, but then suddenly let loose a fiendish yell, as if she were an animal in pain. She continued throwing tape, gowns, and other hospital supplies on the floor, stomping on them when she reached further back to get more. And then, before anyone realized what she was doing, she climbed up onto the shelves, perched on one, and crawled on her hands and knees into the back corner of the shelving, all the while screeching in an unnatural, high-pitched voice, "I . . . want . . . a . . . BEAR . . ."

Dahlia's parents tried to coax her down off the shelf. Then they stretched their arms back to grab her, but the shelf was too deep. Her mother handed her the small bear the volunteer had brought earlier. Dahlia grabbed the bear and threw it like a torpedo right at her mother.

Three adults, one four-year-old, and a stuffed brown bear: a standoff.

"I have to call security," Dr. G told the parents. "I can't let Dahlia hurt herself up there. And I can't let her hurt one of us. I'm sorry. I don't really want to restrain her, but sometimes we have no choice."

Dr. G pushed the door open to summon a security officer. Without warning, Dahlia crawled to the edge of the shelf and jumped off, launching herself at her mother. Her mother caught her and held her tight. With one motion, mother hoisted her back onto the stretcher and hit the power button on the TV with her free hand. Dahlia turned toward the sound of Nemo and the colored pictures flashing on the screen. She looked around and grabbed the stuffed bear, gave it a playful bite on its soft ear, and then hugged it. To everyone's relief, she sat quietly. Soon she was pointing at the screen in delight and laughing at Nemo's antics.

* * *

There is no quick fix for children like Dahlia; no single therapy, medication, emergency room visit, or hospitalization will cure her. She carries a diagnosis of juvenile bipolar disorder, a controversial diagnosis that cannot capture the degree of adversity she has already experienced; it can only describe the constellation of symptoms she demonstrates, which we sometimes call affective or emotional dysregulation. Dahlia suffered so many insults: genetic loading for mental illness, prenatal exposure to drugs and alcohol, early abuse and neglect, and interrupted attachments to primary caregivers. With this list, it is difficult to know where to point the finger or place the blame.

Help for these challenging children comes not from a single intervention but from months and years of interventions. It is a long process fraught with many setbacks and marked by only very gradual forward progress. Children like Dahlia are not one-time visitors to the APS; they are, in ED parlance, frequent flyers. For the staff, it's sometimes difficult to continue to muster the energy or enthusiasm to manage them, particularly when most know that no matter what they do, Dahlia will wreak havoc in the ED, be shipped off to a psychiatric inpatient unit where her medications will be adjusted or changed, be discharged home, and then reappear in the ED within a short period of time to do the whole thing all over again.

Dahlia was admitted to the hospital that day. She was no longer safe to be at home, and her parents understood that safety was the priority. As much as they wanted to bring their daughter home, feed her dinner, and read her a bedtime story, such a pleasant-sounding evening was not in the cards.

Dr. G looked on as Dahlia, now securely strapped to a stretcher for transport, was being loaded into the ambulance.

Her mother stood beside the stretcher, holding Dahlia's little hand. Mother's face was solemn as she turned to Dr. G and said, "I mean this in the nicest way possible, but I hope we never have to see you again."

11

"WE AIN'T NO DELINQUENTS, WE'RE MISUNDERSTOOD"*

"I want him hospitalized," were the first words out of the woman's mouth. She slung her purse over her shoulder and sat down in the chair in front of the triage nurse in the MGH ED. It was 11 P.M.

The "him" in question seemed to be a tall, dark-haired young man wearing wrinkled khaki pants and an equally rumpled button-down shirt, who looked like he had just rolled out of bed. He stood a bit behind his mother with a sheepish grin on his face, flipping his cell phone around in his right hand.

The triage nurse was unfazed. "That will be for the doctors to decide," she said.

The mother opened her bag and started rummaging for something. The young man remained standing, flipping his cell phone and stroking his chin with the other hand as if in deep thought.

"Which one of you is the patient?" the nurse asked.

"He is," the woman said.

"She is," the young man said at the same time.

"Well, who is it?" demanded the triage nurse, "because that person has to sit down and tell me what's going on."

The woman stood up suddenly and gestured to the young man to sit. "He's my son, Steven, and I want him placed in a psychiatric hospital tonight."

Steven smiled at the triage nurse and tried to catch her eye as he slowly tucked his cell phone into his pocket, turned around, and sat down in the chair.

"Your full name, please? And your date of birth?" she asked. Appearing somewhat indifferent to the answers, she placed his right arm in the blood pressure cuff, captured his right forefinger in a pulse oximeter, and, at the same time, in one smooth, well-practiced movement, ran the thermometer over his forehead. Beep—the machine registered Steven's normal blood pressure, heart rate, and oxygen saturation. He had no fever.

---

*"Gee, Officer Krupke," *West Side Story,* Sondheim and Bernstein.

"You're Steven, you're 16, and I gather that your mother thinks you need psychiatric help," said the triage nurse as she gestured to one of the security guards to call the APS resident to come and evaluate the situation a bit further. "Any medical problems?" she continued.

"Nope."

"Do you take any medications?"

"Nope."

"Allergic to anything?"

"Nope."

"Use drugs or alcohol?"

"Nope."

"Do you think you need psychiatric help?"

"Of course not," he said, sitting back in the chair, crossing his legs, and absentmindedly rubbing a small, round scar on his left forearm. "I'm fine."

"You thinking of hurting yourself or anyone else?"

"Never have."

"What's the scar from?" she pointed to his arm.

"Nothing. A friend tried to stab me with a pen to wake me up."

Before Steven had a chance to elaborate, the APS resident came around the corner.

The triage nurse gave her the little information she had and shrugged her shoulders.

The resident turned to Steven's mother. "Tell me what's happening here."

"Doctor, there is something wrong with my son; he definitely has a piece missing. He doesn't listen. He acts on impulse. He can't tell right from wrong. He needs to be evaluated by a psychiatrist, a good psychiatrist. We were in court today and the judge told me that Steven must have an inpatient admission," she said. "Preferably at this hospital," she added. "He's been other places but they weren't any good."

"So here we are," Steven chimed in, as if his statement of the obvious was all that needed to be said on the matter.

The resident found it very unlikely that a judge had mandated a psychiatric evaluation at 11 P.M. with the goal of having Steven admitted electively to MGH, but she didn't point that out. If Steven had indeed been in court that day and the judge had wanted a psychiatric evaluation, he could have requested that one be done on-site by a specially trained psychologist. Steven was too young to be admitted to the adult inpatient med-psych unit on site at the MGH; the unit was only for adults. Furthermore, the fact that Steven had a history of psychiatric hospitalizations suggested that there might be something more than a missing piece going on.

She also knew that the waiting room was full, and Steven seemed just a bit edgy, so even though he had denied any safety issues, she decided to secure him in one of the holding rooms. Clearly, there was more to this story, but it would have to wait until someone had time to sort it out. In the meantime, she ordered a urine toxicology screen—every patient with "teen" in the number of his age got such a screen. If it came back negative for drugs of abuse—no harm done. If it were positive, it would be enlightening.

It was about 2 A.M. when the on-call resident had time to find out why Steven and his mother had picked this particular night to show up in the APS. This may be the most important question to ask when beginning a psychiatric evaluation in an emergency room: What makes this day or night different from all others? In other words, why did this patient show up at this time on this day? There is always a reason, and usually the reason is relevant.

In Steven's case, the story emerged slowly and painfully.

With adolescents, it's usually better to interview the patient first before getting further information from the parent (or other caregiver with legal custody). Adolescents are usually in the process of trying to separate themselves from their parents or caregivers. By allowing the teen to tell his or her own story first, the interviewer, whether resident, nurse, social worker, or medical student, can respect this developmentally appropriate desire for autonomy. This does not mean that the evaluator can forgo talking with everyone else involved in the adolescent's life. Collateral information is always crucial. However, offering the teenager the option to tell his or her story to a nonprejudiced listener can be a good way to encourage disclosure.

Teenagers often want to know if what they tell the clinician will be held in confidence. Unfortunately, in a hospital ED, few things remain confidential. Anyone under the age of 18 is considered a minor in the eyes of the law, and legal guardians (usually parents) have the right to request a copy of a minor child's medical records. Even though according to Massachusetts law (General Laws, Chapter 112, Section 12f) it is not necessary to obtain the consent of a parent or legal guardian for treatment if the minor is married, widowed or divorced, already a parent, pregnant, enlisted in the armed forces, living separately and managing his or her finances, or suffering from a sexually transmitted infection (STI), most of the time, parents and/or guardians are informed about their child's presence in the ED and his or her care. Generally speaking, most of what happens in the APS will filter back to the parents. Unless the teen fits into one of the categories listed previously, the parents can obtain laboratory results including pregnancy tests and toxicology screens. Certainly, if the teen's life (or someone else's life) is at risk, the parents must be told.

Drawing on what she remembered about adolescent development, the senior resident decided to interview Steven alone before talking with his mother. Steven had fallen asleep on the stretcher; his mother was sound asleep beside him on another stretcher that had been moved into the holding room. Despite the fact that she wanted her son admitted to a psychiatric hospital because she didn't feel safe taking him home, she apparently also felt unwilling to leave him alone in the ED, even for a few hours.

Interviewing a very young child in the middle of the night can often be less than helpful. Most small children are sleepy and irritable, and it is often impossible to speak with any of their outpatient caregivers by phone in order to supplement the picture. Sometimes sleep therapy is more valuable; if a child has fallen asleep in a holding room, letting him or her rest until the morning may be best for all concerned. This runs counter to procedure in most EDs, which is to evaluate, treat, and discharge as quickly as possible. Nevertheless, for young children who present with psychiatric issues, it is often wiser (and even necessary) to wait and gather more history in the morning.

But teenagers are different. They can manage a middle of the night evaluation. So the resident woke Steven up to talk with him, asking the mother to return to the waiting room while Steven told his version of the story.

It was all a matter of misunderstanding, Steven began. His parents were divorced several years ago, and he currently lived south of Boston with his mother, 14-year-old brother, and two much younger brothers who were still in elementary school. His father lived nearby, and the kids went back and forth between their parents' houses, but they mostly stayed with their mother because their dad drank too much and his ex-wife didn't approve. Steven himself didn't have any kind of psychiatric problems, but he thought his mother was too anxious and his brother was "crazy." He and his brother frequently got into scrapes. Four days earlier, the two had been drinking and wrestling in the living room, and somehow a brass candlestick had fallen off the mantelpiece and hit the brother's head. When Steven saw that his brother was bleeding profusely from his scalp, he called 911. But when the police showed up at the house, they took his brother to the hospital and arrested Steven. He had spent four days in juvenile detention before the judge had released him to his mother's custody. He wasn't sure what type of psychiatric care the judge had demanded, but he didn't think he needed much. He was willing to do some outpatient substance abuse counseling to please the court. He was sure he didn't need anything else; he wasn't depressed or anything like that. After he got out of court, he and his mother had gone home because he really wanted to shower, change, and have something good to eat. The other kids were at their father's house.

"And then she made me come here," he finished.

"Anyone worried about you and your brother going at it again?" asked the resident.

"Nah. We were just wrestling. He didn't even get knocked out. He just got some stitches this time. He's fine."

"Are you worried about being in trouble with the law?"

"I don't see why you are making a big deal about this."

"What big deal?"

"I didn't hurt anyone."

"I get it. I get it. You didn't hurt anyone. So why did you tell the judge you would agree to outpatient drug counseling? I thought I heard you tell the triage nurse that you didn't use drugs."

"I stopped a few months ago. It's not a problem."

"Why did your friend have to stab you with a pen to wake you up?"

"Whatever. I was out of it."

"What kinds of drugs do you use?"

"I've tried a lot of stuff."

"Like what?"

"Oh, weed. Tried coke a few times. Maybe some Ecstasy."

"Benzos?"

"If they were around."

"Like what?"

"I don't know, like Valium, Xanax, that kind of stuff."

"IV drugs?"

"Never."

"Alcohol?"

"I quit drinking."

"How much could you put away?"

"Like 5–6 beers and a couple of shots."

"Every day?"

Steven gave her a look that was almost a sneer. "When I could find it."

"Ever have blackouts? Hallucinations? Seizures?"

Steven didn't answer.

"OK, when was your last drink?" The resident needed to know if Steven was at risk for the potentially life-threatening alcohol withdrawal syndrome that can affect daily drinkers two to three days after they stop cold turkey. She thought about giving him the CRAFFT screening (self-report questionnaire for adolescents about substance use and associated behavior patterns) but figured she'd lose him if she took that path. It was clear that Steven wouldn't be leaving the APS any time soon and that she would have plenty of time later to fill in the picture. There were already too many unanswered questions, and the evaluation was beginning to sound like a distorted game of Clue with who used the candlestick in the living room.

"I don't drink. I told you. The police arrested me because I've been on probation for months."

The resident shifted gears. "Probation for what?"

"Tried to lift some stuff from a Best Buy. But I didn't mean anything by it. It was on a dare. They got me for B & E."

"Do you have a probation officer?"

"Yeah. Bill somebody. My mother has the information. She's the whole reason I'm here. I mean, I have to get this court problem settled, but there is nothing else going on."

"Nothing else? Your mother said something about you having been in some psychiatric hospitals before."

"I was tricked. I hurt my arm a few weeks ago and the docs in the ED from another hospital sent me to some shit-hole unit. I signed a three-day and they let me out."

"Docs don't usually send kids to psychiatric hospitals for arm pain. Is there more to the story?"

"Not really. The psych unit let me go, didn't they? I'm not dangerous to anyone. Can I have my cell phone back?"

"You have an important call to make?"

"My girlfriend."

"Where is she?"

"I assume she's at home." Steven turned away from the resident and buried his face in the pillow. "I've got nothing more to say," his voice muffled and indistinct. "Just talk to my mother, if you want. I need some sleep."

Apparently the interview was over. The resident told the APS nurse that Steven could have his cell phone and went in search of Mrs. Y.

"Urine tox positive for marijuana, nothing else," the nurse reported as she headed out to the waiting room.

The mother was sleeping in one of the chairs with her head on her arm. The resident shook her gently, and she jerked awake.

"Sorry," she said. "I just closed my eyes for a minute. It's been a long day." She followed the resident into one of the interview rooms, trying to smooth her hair and straighten her shirt as she went.

Mrs. Y's blustery manner was all but gone. She spoke quietly and offered a slightly different account of recent events. Steven was always a really smart kid. He was diagnosed with attention hyperactivity deficit disorder (ADHD) when he was in the third grade. He took stimulants for a while as prescribed by his pediatrician and had some outpatient counseling, but he never really clicked with anyone. However, he was so impulsive and distractible that even with medication he was a serious management problem in the classroom; he picked fights with other kids and stole things from family members and friends. When he was 13, he started drinking and smoking pot. By the time he started high school, his substance use had escalated to include cocaine, opiates, and hallucinogens. His parents didn't know what to do with him. Eventually, they sent him to a wilderness program for a few months followed by placement in a therapeutic boarding school in yet another state for teens with behavioral problems. Finally, he returned home just before he turned 16 to start his sophomore year at the local public high school.

Trouble with the law started right away. Six months ago, he and his younger brother stole their grandmother's car, took it out for a joyride, and ended up stuck in mud in a deep ditch on the side of a highway. Luckily, no one was hurt. This was the beginning of a downward spiral that involved four or five legal entanglements for drug possession, and petty theft, and several brief psychiatric hospitalizations, culminating in the arrest for breaking and entering. The court placed him on probation and sent him to a day program for teens with substance abuse issues, but after completing only a week of the program, he said he didn't find it helpful and refused to go back. More recently, he had fallen down a set of stairs while intoxicated. He thought he was fine, but when he complained of some arm pain the next morning, his mother brought him to a local ED. While there, she asked for a psychiatric evaluation because she was worried that his fall had been a suicide attempt even though Steven vehemently denied wanting to hurt himself in any way. After a few hours in that ED, he tried to escape and was restrained and medicated before being committed on a Section 12 to an inpatient psychiatric unit on the grounds of his inability to care for himself.

"He said he signed out of the unit after 72 hours," the resident interjected.

"Yes, that's right. They said they couldn't keep him because he wasn't dangerous to himself or to anyone else. That's always how it is."

"What about the fall?"

"He said it was an accident."

Mother's phone buzzed, and she glanced at it. "I bet that's a text from Steven."

"Is it?"

She read, 'Something inside me is going to snap if I go to an inpatient unit.'

The phone buzzed again and she continued, "If you don't let me come home, I will kill you." "That's Steven for you." She laughed without meaning it.

"You think he will hurt you?"

"No. He never has. He hasn't ever hurt anyone. He's not really aggressive. He just doesn't know his limits."

"Should we take his phone away? If we confiscate his phone, he won't send you any more texts like that."

"No. It's fine." She seemed resigned.

"What about his brother and the candlestick?"

"I know it sounds ridiculous, but it is very plausible that my other son was hurt by accident; the two of them are always going at it."

"So you believe their story?"

"Actually, yes. I believe Steven's right on this one."

"But you want Steven in the hospital again?"

"I can't have him coming back to the house until he gets treatment. There is definitely something wrong. I told you before—he has some kind of piece missing. This kid is really smart. He wants to go to college. He went to a therapeutic school, he has been to psych hospitals and to wilderness programs. Nothing has helped. The mental health system is broken."

"So what do you think he needs now?"

"I think he needs to be admitted to MGH."

"He can't be admitted here, it's a unit for adults. He's too young."

"Well, then admit him to the best unit for teenagers."

"Why do you think another inpatient stay will be any different than his previous inpatient experiences?"

"If he can't get help from whatever you think is the best unit, I just give up."

"What happens if he doesn't go to a hospital?"

"Well, I don't want him locked up in juvenile detention again—that's just jail. The judge thought about that today, or maybe it was yesterday by this time, but then I talked with him and he decided Steven really needed more psychiatric help."

"Do you think that his stays on psych units have helped him?"

"It's better than letting him get himself into trouble. I can't get him to go to outpatient care; I can't take him home. I have younger children."

"I'm not sure he's really committable—"

She interrupted the resident. "Not committable? Not committable? Steven drinks, he uses drugs, he is really impulsive and he acts on instinct. Now he's facing an assault and battery charge 'cause of that fight with his brother. He is on probation and supposed to be sober, and then he ends up in that hospital ED after he got so drunk he fell down a set of stairs. Bet he has drugs in his system today—probation or no probation. The next thing I know, the state will be after me for keeping Steven at home because those case workers will think that he poses a danger to my other kids. And I don't want to have a run-in with the state; I don't want to lose my little boys."

"But he's not dangerous to himself or others."

"What about the text I just read you?"

"But you told me you weren't afraid of him, that he just says things like that to get attention but doesn't mean them. You didn't even want me to take his phone away."

Mrs. Y sat and stared at the resident. "You're just like all the others," she said. "I'm telling you that there is something wrong, something seriously wrong, and you're telling me that you can't help my son. He's 16 now. He's going to be 18 in less than two years. Once he turns 18, he's a goner, he'll just go to jail."

"I understand it's a tough situation. But Steven doesn't want to be admitted and I can't force him into a psych unit against his will. Hasn't helped him much before. I can refer him for outpatient substance abuse treatment if you like."

"Outpatient substance abuse treatment for a kid who has never been willing to admit that he has a substance abuse problem? A kid who says he hasn't had a drink in months and then two weeks ago falls down a set of stairs drunk as a skunk? You have got to be kidding me. He just smooth-talks his way out of everything. He knows just what to say." She paused and sat back in her chair. "If you were in my shoes, what would you do?"

* * *

What should the APS resident do?

Let's review the history. Steven carries the diagnosis of ADHD; his inattention, impulsivity, and hyperactivity got him into trouble both at home and at school. He took stimulants when he was young, but it is not clear whether they helped him. He also meets criteria for conduct disorder (CD) given his level of aggression and violence, his stealing, and his use of weapons. (Only his mother believes that the brother's scalp laceration was caused by a candlestick that fell from the mantelpiece and does not blame Steven for what happened.) In addition, he definitely has problems with alcohol and drugs and continues to make risky decisions, particularly when under the influence.

Does Steven have an emerging antisocial personality disorder?

Children with CD are at high risk for developing delinquency in adulthood. Some data from magnetic resonance imagery studies suggest that the brains of boys with CD and ADHD show changes that look like those seen in the brains of antisocial adults.[1] Would it be fair to say that Steven's neurobiology predisposes him to behave in ways that are socially maladaptive? Will he become a sociopath simply because he is wired that way, because it is in his nature?

And what about other psychological or social risk factors for delinquency? His parents are divorced, and his father drinks too much. Steven thinks his mother is anxious and his brother is crazy. We don't know much about his relationships with his friends and whether he hangs with a tough crowd. Did he witness violence at home? Was he abused himself? Does he have a mood or anxiety disorder that he is self-medicating with alcohol and drugs? In other words, does Steven's disruptive behavior stem from emotional problems? He did not appear to be depressed or anxious on the night he showed up in the emergency room, but could his insolence and provocative comments simply cover up his poor self-esteem and intense neediness? Does he have an as-yet-undiagnosed psychiatric problem that needs treatment? Is he indeed just misunderstood?

Even if Steven's difficulties can best be characterized as a consequence of that complex dance between nature and nurture, how does that understanding change our management? Yes, Steven is a juvenile offender, but perhaps there is still hope for rehabilitation. Should the resident stretch the limits and send Steven to yet another psychiatric hospital using that imprecise third criteria for commitment—"inability to care for self," even if it is extremely likely that if she commits him, he will just behave himself and sign out within three days, as he has done several times before? So, forget rehabilitation—should Steven face the consequences of his actions and potentially be incarcerated for his behavior? Should she discharge him home with his mother and let the chips fall where they may? Steven is not actively dangerous to himself. He is not professing suicidal ideation, plan, or intent. He claims the scar on his arm was made by a friend because he was so out of it that his buddies couldn't think of another way to wake him up. He denies ever having meant to hurt anyone else. Nevertheless, the chance that he will continue to violate his probation and end up back in juvenile detention or in jail remains high. Does he deserve that?

Unfortunately, there is no right answer to these questions—there is only the answer that seems right at the time.

On that night, Steven steadfastly maintained that he was willing to accept some outpatient help—but only because it would make him look better in court. So, after consultation with the attending physician, the resident scheduled an appointment for 10 days later at a local outpatient program specializing in substance abuse issues that was geared to adolescents, young adults, and their families. Then she discharged Steven, and he went home with his mother.

* * *

One week later, Steven and his mother returned to the APS, again with his mother demanding hospitalization. She reported that over the past week, Steven had had several angry outbursts and become verbally but not physically abusive toward her. She was worried that he was going to do something stupid and get into trouble with the law. Again, Steven was on his best behavior; he denied any safety issues and did not send any provocative text messages. The staff was annoyed. This mother–son duo was singing the same tune; nothing had changed. Steven thought his mother was foolish; he still didn't think he needed any help at all. The APS clinicians thought: what a waste of resources. Time, energy, effort—all for a kid who couldn't care less. Again he was discharged home with a plan to keep the outpatient appointment with the substance abuse clinic that had been scheduled at the time of his first APS visit and to check in with his probation officer as ordered by the court.

* * *

The pair returned a third time two days later. Mrs. Y was extremely upset because Steven had gone missing and later been found at a friend's house asleep on the pool table. He had had too much to drink, passed out, and missed his curfew. Although his mother was worried that the judge would now send Steven to juvenile detention for violation of his probation, Steven himself was not worried.

"I'll just hitchhike to California," he told the resident who saw him that night.

Once more, the APS resident offered Steven the option of elective admission to an inpatient psychiatric unit or discharge to home, stressing the risk of more time in juvenile detention should he continue to violate the conditions of probation.

This time, Steven chose the psychiatric unit.

Did he choose to enter treatment because he had a glimmer of insight into his own situation and was finally ready to take a look at his own actions, or did he just think that going inpatient would look better in court? Who knows?

* * *

Steven signed out of the inpatient psychiatric unit with the consent of his mother but against medical advice after a few days.

Note

1. Heubner T, Vloet T, Marx I, Konrad K, Fink G, Herphertz S, Herphertz-Dahlmann B. Morphometric brain abnormalities in boys with conduct disorder. *J Am Acad Child Adolesc Psychiatry* 2008 57(5): 540–547.

12

SUICIDE BY SECURITY BLANKET

At 10 P.M., the child psychiatry resident called her attending, Dr. T, to ask for help. "We have a nine-year-old kid here, Tommy, who is suicidal and his mother doesn't seem to get it. The kid tried to strangle himself earlier today and she's saying that we're making this up and that her son is not in crisis. She is all ready to take him home. What am I supposed to do?"

"Where is the nine-year-old now?" Dr. T asked her.

"He's sitting in an interview room. His mother is on the phone with his father in another interview room yelling that it's all Tommy's fault. She's blaming the kid for the problem. This kid needs to be hospitalized. He's the real deal."

"Did he hurt his neck when he tried to strangle himself? Has anyone actually looked at him?"

"Pediatrics saw him just a few minutes ago after he told us what he had done. They said his neck was fine. He didn't need cervical spine films. Can we commit the kid against the parents' wishes?"

"Yes, we can," the attending replied, "as long as we have grounds to do so. Put the kid in a holding room and have security tell mother she needs to wait. Fill out a Section 12. He's committable on the grounds of dangerousness to self. I will be right in."

* * *

There are very few reasons that an attending child psychiatrist has to come in to the ED at night: committing a minor to a locked inpatient unit against the will of the parents or guardians is one of them. There is an adult attending psychiatrist physically in the APS until 10 P.M., and there are two adult psychiatry residents (one junior, one senior) who work overnight. The child psychiatry residents take call as well, and one is always available 24/7. Generally, on nights and weekends, the adult residents page the child psychiatry residents to "run the child case by them," and then the child psychiatry resident pages the child psych attending on call that week to review the case and formulate both

a diagnosis and a disposition before calling the adult resident back to implement the plan. Sometimes the system is cumbersome—there can be a time lag
while waiting for one or another doc to return a page—but usually it works.
MGH is a teaching hospital; residents need a chance to air the details and to
think out loud with someone who has more experience before committing
themselves or a patient and family to a course of action. Sometimes, though,
the issues are just too complex to be managed by remote control.

* * *

Dr. E, the child psychiatry resident on call that night, had come in to interview Tommy and his family members. As soon as she arrived, one of the
nurses came over to her waving some white papers.

"Here's what the mother gave us at triage," she said. "We made some copies. Looks like this kid is pretty depressed. He made a couple of lists about why
he should or should not kill himself."

Dr. E glanced down at the pages. Tommy had written on the top of the page
"LIST OF WHY I WANT TO DIE." Underneath, he had written a long list of
the reasons that he should be dead including: Nobody cares about me; I have
no friends; I am BAD; No one will notice.

"Pretty clear what he had in mind," Dr. E said.

"Yeah. I had security put the mother in an interview room. She wasn't help-
ing the kid one bit, just telling him to keep his mouth shut or we would lock
him up. Now she's on the phone with someone."

"I called Dr. T and he's coming in," Dr. E told the nurse. "This could get
messy. Kid has to go into the hospital, don't you think?"

"This kid is scared of his own shadow. Most fourth graders don't carry
around a security blanket. Kid's in there clutching his. It's pretty dirty and it
looks like he wiped his nose with it, but whatever."

"I guess I'll go in to see him. Sounds like a sad guy. Maybe Dr. T will deal
with the mother."

"That mother's a piece of work," the nurse said.

* * *

Dr. E went into Bay 40 to talk with Tommy. He was small for his age and
slightly chubby with curly black hair. His face was smudged with dirt, and he
had clearly been crying. He sat cross-legged on the stretcher close to one end,
holding the sheet up around his neck.

A nursing assistant sat quietly in a corner, watching.

Dr. E went to stand at the foot of the stretcher and smiled as she faced
Tommy. "Hi," she said. "How are you doing?"

"I'm OK." His voice was just a shade louder than a whisper, but he looked
directly at her. The expression on his face did not change.

Dr. E stopped smiling. "I heard that you have been thinking of hurting yourself."

"I hate myself. I want to die." Tommy's voice lacked any inflection.

"Why?"

"I'm bad. The world is bad. No one likes me. No one wants me as a friend."

"No one?"

"I'm a loser. No one wants to be friends with a loser. They all hate me."

"Why are you a loser?"

"I'm fat. I can't do anything right. I got into trouble at school."

"What happened at school?"

"Nothing."

"Nothing?"

"I wrote some bad stuff."

"Bad stuff?"

"This one kid farts all the time and I wrote 'fart' on his notebook."

"Then what happened?"

"The teacher made me apologize."

"That's it?"

"My parents get mad when I do stuff like that."

"Were they mad this time?"

"I don't know. I always get in trouble. No one in my family likes me, either. They won't care if I'm dead."

"So after what happened in school you started to think about killing yourself?"

"I think about it a lot."

"You do?"

He nodded.

"When do you think those thoughts?"

"A lot."

"Tell me."

"When I do something bad. When I mess up."

"Mess up?"

"You know, when I fight with my sister, or lose something, or tell a lie. When I get mad at myself it just makes sense."

"What makes sense?"

"It's really the only option for me."

"Have you ever tried to kill yourself before this?"

"Not really," he said.

"Well." Dr. E paused before asking, "What happened this time?"

"My mother caught me before I could do it," he muttered.

"What happened?"

Tommy's voice got just a bit louder. "After school, I was really mad. I went down to the playroom and I tried to strangle myself. I didn't have any rope, so I used my scarf. I also thought about going upstairs and trying to jump out a window."

"Did you hurt yourself when you tied the scarf around your neck?"

"No. I couldn't get it that tight."

"Did you think that you could kill yourself that way?"

"If I pulled hard enough."

"So what happened then?"

"My mother came downstairs and found me."

"I guess it was lucky that your mother was keeping an eye on you. Do you know why she came down?"

"I don't know. She took the scarf away and called the doctor. Here's the scarf." Tommy pushed the sheet away from him. He was wearing maroon hospital PJ's that were slightly too big for him. Around his neck hung a dirty grey-colored knit scarf that looked as if it might once have been another color, perhaps light blue. It had remnants of fringe hanging from each end. The scarf hung loosely, and the ends tumbled into his lap. As he spoke, Tommy absent-mindedly started stroking the tattered fringe on one end.

Dr. E tried to regroup. How could the nurses have let this kid sit in a bay with a scarf around his neck when apparently he had just tried to strangle himself with that very scarf?

"Is this the same scarf?" she asked him.

"Yes. I just told you that. I had it with me."

"Is this scarf your 'security blanket'? Do you sleep with it?" Dr. E hoped she didn't sound quite as incredulous as she felt.

"Well, I don't take it to school, usually. It usually stays on my bed during the day." He paused before adding, "I had it with me today. It was in my backpack. It used to be light blue. I've had it for as long as I can remember. I think my father gave it to my mother but she didn't like it."

"You tried to strangle yourself with the scarf you have held on to forever?"

Tommy was silent.

Dr. E fell silent, too.

Somewhat awkwardly, Tommy again began stroking the end of his scarf. He looked at her. "Are you going to take it away?" His voice shook just slightly.

Dr. E was at a loss. Should she take the scarf away? If Tommy had been three years old, this would have been a different story. Toddlers often carry special blankets or pillows or stuffed animals for comfort when they face a stressful situation or a separation. But at age nine, Tommy was too old to be carrying a security blanket around with him. Furthermore, kids in holding rooms weren't allowed to have anything that they could use to harm them-selves. But if she took the scarf away, would Tommy feel worse? Should she ask him if he would let her hold on to it for safekeeping? Should she demand that he give it up? Maybe she could get away with letting him keep it if he took it off his neck. He did have a nursing assistant sitting with him. If he tried to tighten the scarf around his neck, she would be there to intervene.

"Seems like this scarf is really important to you," she said slowly.

Tommy nodded.

"Any chance you'd be willing just to hold that scarf in your lap while you're here?" she asked him. "I don't want to have to take the scarf away."

"OK," he said, and he slowly slid the scarf off his neck and tucked it under his legs. "Is it OK if I take a nap?"

"Of course," she said. "You must be tired; it's late."

Tommy lay down on the stretcher, reached back, and shifted his tangled scarf so that it bunched up under his chin. Dr. E helped him to pull the sheet up around his shoulders. He closed his eyes.

* * *

"Did you know that this kid tried to strangle himself with the same scarf he has draped around his neck?" she asked the nurse sitting outside the bay as soon as she had shut the door behind her.

"I thought that might be it," said the nurse. "But it's his 'blankie'—what was I going to do, take away the object that brings him comfort? He has company now; the nursing assistant is in there. I wouldn't have left him alone, but I didn't see hurting him further."

"I had the same thought," Dr. E said. "No right answer there."

The nurse nodded. "He's just a kid."

"Where's his mother?" Dr. E asked.

"Can't you hear her?"

"She's the woman yelling?"

"That's her." Dr. E went around the corner and saw Tommy's mother standing in an interview room gesticulating with her right hand while holding the telephone to her ear with her left hand. She was casually dressed, wearing dark pants and a white blouse with a brightly colored silk scarf tucked in at the collar. She slammed the receiver down just as Dr. E approached the door.

"What is it?" the mother asked Dr. E.

"I'm Dr. E, the child psychiatry resident. Do you mind if we talk?"

"There is nothing to talk about. Our pediatrician sent Tommy here. I called him this afternoon after I found Tommy trying to tighten that silly scarf he wears around his neck. The pediatrician insisted that I bring him right in here. But nothing, absolutely nothing has happened. We have been here for hours. I just spoke with my husband. My other kids are still up. I need to go home to put them to bed. Everything is just a mess."

"What were you expecting when you brought Tommy here?"

"I was not expecting that he would be sitting around in a room by himself for hours. I know he's upset, he's been talking about killing himself for the past few months. I showed the nurse the new list I found. But he's always writing something and leaving it out for me to see. Sometimes he leaves little notes in my purse: 'I'm a loser' or 'Bad boy' or 'Better off dead.' But he's never done anything to hurt himself."

"Until today," Dr. E interjected.

"When he came home from school, he didn't look right," mother continued. "I just knew something was up. He went right downstairs to the playroom and usually he has something to eat first thing. So I followed him down there."

"Were you frightened?"

"Frightened? No." She sat down heavily in one of the chairs, but Dr. E remained standing in the doorway. "Frankly, I just think he should get over it already. We have a beautiful home. I don't know what Tommy is so upset about. We even got him someone to talk to a few weeks ago, but it didn't work out because our insurance wouldn't cover the doctor's visits."

"I didn't know Tommy had an outpatient doctor."

"He doesn't. That's what he needs, I guess. He only saw this therapist once. I take it back—he saw him once and we saw him once."

"Did you try to find someone who is in your insurance network?"

"We filed an appeal with the insurer because Tommy seemed to like the therapist, but it didn't go through. We just got word about that," she sighed.

"Did he talk to the therapist about feeling suicidal?"

"Oh. Yes. That's what he was there for, right? I think the therapist was worried. But we were watching him and he was just fine. That's when he wrote those lists I gave the nurse."

"He wrote those a few weeks ago?"

"Yes. I told you, he's always writing something like that."

"Was today the first time he ever tried to hurt himself?"

"I wouldn't exactly call it hurting himself."

"Was today the first time he tied his scarf around his neck?"

"As far as I know. He carries that scarf everywhere. He'd take it to school, but a few years ago I told him he couldn't because the other kids would laugh at him. Now he leaves it at home under his pillow. At least he says he does. But we really need to get home. My husband will be upset if we don't get home soon. I told you, I have younger children, and they need me. We just need some kind of outpatient doctor—someone who will take our insurance."

"Mrs. D," Dr. E began, "I think that Tommy needs more than outpatient care right now. He needs to be in the hospital."

"What are you talking about, young lady? That is simply ridiculous. You are obviously not a mother. No mother would let her kid be locked up on a psych ward." Tommy's mother stood up again and started to head for the door.

"Please don't leave the room," Dr. E said.

"I have a beautiful home. I have a husband. I have two other children. Tommy is fine."

"We're worried that he could really hurt himself given the way he is feeling now."

"I'll take that chance."

"But we can't," Dr. E heard a pleading tone creep into her voice. "Psychiatric hospitals are not terrible places. Your son will be safe on an inpatient unit. He can get some help there. I called my supervisor, Dr. T. He's on his way in to the hospital. I think you'll have to talk with him. Tommy is pretty troubled."

"You call your supervisor. I'm calling my husband and my lawyer."

* * *

Dr. E went back to the room where the on-call residents were busy working, leaving the mother to her phone calls.

"Mother's calling her attorney," she explained to the adult psychiatry attending sitting there. "She kept telling me that she has a beautiful home. I can't imagine. Did you know that the kid is in the holding room cuddling with the same scarf he tied around his neck earlier today? I guess I have to call the hospital lawyer and alert whoever is on call in the Office of General Counsel that this patient's mother is really upset."

"Did you offer to have a rep from 'patient advocacy' come by to talk with her?" the other doctor asked.

"I think they're only here during the day. And I don't think this mother would agree, anyway."

"You should still offer."

A nurse came in. "Can I let the mother back in with Tommy? He's fast asleep, but she's asking to go back in to sit with him."

Dr. E shrugged. "I don't see why not."

Dr. T arrived and listened to Dr. E's story.

"The mother is calling her husband and her lawyer now?" he asked. "Well, I'll try to reason with her. Did you file a 51A with DCF?"

"File with DCF?"

"Yes. You have to. Basically, you're telling me that the parents have been ignoring their nine-year-old who has been dropping notes in his mother's purse saying he'll be better off dead. Is that right? And the parents didn't follow up with the outpatient provider? Did anyone call that therapist?"

"One of the adult residents."

"What did he say?"

"Kid came once; parents came once. Insurance didn't work out. Never heard from them again."

"Did the kid tell the therapist he was suicidal?"

"Yes, but the therapist thought the parents were following up with someone who took their insurance."

"Really? Did he check?" Dr. T paused. "Don't answer that. I don't want to know. But we definitely file on the parents. This is neglect. They knew that their kid was thinking about killing himself but they didn't get him any help? And now you're telling me that they refuse to allow him to be hospitalized. They think they can manage him? Or maybe they are just afraid of what he might say about life with them. Some beautiful home, huh?"

The nurse came back in. "Mother's losing it," she said. "Can't you hear her from here?"

"What's she saying?" Dr. T asked.

"She woke her son up and started yelling at him. 'See what you did? Did you get what you wanted? It's all your fault that they are taking you away from me,'" the nurse parroted in a high pitched voice full of anger. "Can I have security put her back in the waiting room?"

"Have them take her out of there but put her in an interview room. I'll meet with her now," Dr. T said.

* * *

Dr. T, a big man wearing a slightly rumpled blue blazer, sat down in one of the chairs and motioned for Tommy's mother to join him. He rested his elbow on the desk and leaned back slightly as he gently explained that the hospital staff planned to hospitalize her son and also to file a report with DCF for alleged neglect.

"My husband is at home and our attorney is on the phone with him now. The lawyer says you can't do this. We are Tommy's parents; we decide what happens."

"Mrs. D, I have a duty to hospitalize your son and I can do it against your will. I prefer not to. I think we both want to help your son to feel better."

"Locking him up in a mental ward won't help."

"Hear me out. Whatever is happening with him—it's serious. And for whatever reason, he hasn't gotten better, he's gotten worse. There's no way you can keep an eye on him every minute; what would have happened if you hadn't followed him downstairs to the playroom this afternoon? Let's keep him safe while we're trying to figure out what is wrong. This will also give us time to set up some outpatient care so that when he leaves the hospital, he'll have someone looking out for him in a way that's different than what you can do."

"I think you are blowing this situation all out of proportion."

"Maybe we are. But maybe we're not. I heard that you told my resident you were willing to take a chance with Tommy. I am not."

"And what if I refuse?" She glared at him.

"Then I have security escort you off the premises and I send Tommy to the psychiatric hospital without you," Dr. T said. He let a few seconds go by before adding, "But we don't have to do it that way."

For a few minutes, neither of them said anything. Mrs. D sat with her hands on her knees, staring at the floor. Dr. T remained in the same position he was in before, legs crossed, elbow resting on the desk, and head on his hand.

"Where are you sending him and when?" she finally blurted out.

"Unfortunately, I don't really know the answer to either question," Dr. T replied. "This is an emergency department—it's a busy, complicated place. Not ideal for you or for your son. I am sorry about that. Arranging for an inpatient psychiatric hospitalization will take a little time. I have to find an open bed and then I have to get your insurance company to agree with my assessment and pre-certify his admission. He'll probably be here overnight."

"Here? In this pit? Overnight?"

"You can stay with him if you want. He'll be safe here."

"Then I insist on taking him home."

"I can't let you do that."

Mrs. D turned her head away. "Well, then you talk to my husband and explain why I can't bring Tommy home. He won't believe me. And you'd better call your lawyer in the morning because my husband is not going to let you get away with this."

"Is your husband planning to come in to the ED? I'd be happy to talk with him, too."

"You ask him," she said. "I'm finished."

* * *

Tommy did spend the night in the ED, just as Dr. T had predicted. His insurance company approved three days' inpatient hospitalization with review for additional days, but there were no beds available in the middle of the night. His mother stayed with him overnight. In the morning, his father arrived and sat silently with his son and wife in the holding room. No one mentioned legal action. Eventually, the resource specialist found an open inpatient bed, the nurses called for an ambulance, and the EMTs arrived to pick up Tommy to take him to his next hospital.

And what about the scarf? When housekeeping came to clean the holding room after Tommy left, the janitor found it under the sheet on the stretcher in the holding room. The nurses held on to it for a few days, but no one came to claim it and finally someone tossed it.

Afterword

Between 50 and 75 children cross the APS threshold every month. Yet the MGH is not unique. Nationwide, it is more and more common for emergency department clinicians to serve as mental health providers for those children and families who have fallen through multiple safety nets. Most of these patients cannot obtain help anywhere else due to acute shortages of inpatient and residential beds, child psychiatrists and other qualified caregivers, as well as limitations on insurance coverage for what is euphemistically called "behavioral health." The tales in this collection open the door to this hidden world—a locked pod tucked deep within a major metropolitan hospital's emergency room, a place to which many children and families turn when there is nowhere else to go.

One of the most difficult aspects of working in an ED is that one rarely learns what happens to the patient after he or she leaves. Disposition is not treatment. Once the patient has been stabilized, emergency room doctors—internists or pediatricians, surgeons or psychiatrists—usually find themselves asking the same questions: Can the patient go home? Does the patient need to be admitted to the hospital? Answering these questions allows us to determine where the patient goes next—what happens after that will be someone else's job.

In general, child psychiatrists in the ED do not stare into crystal balls or read tea leaves. Instead, we carefully gather as much detail as possible—the psychiatric history—and make our decisions based on our interpretation of the data. Despite our best intentions, we run the risk of sending a potentially suicidal child home or sending a vulnerable child to an inpatient hospital where he or she feels endangered rather than safe. Sometimes we make poor choices based on incomplete information; sometimes the children and families themselves prevent us from doing what we think may be in their best interest. Yet we muddle on, trusting that we will be able to offer most of our patients the acute care and attention they need and then help them to plan for what lies ahead.

In the end, that is the most difficult lesson: those of us who care for children under these circumstances must learn to live with uncertainty. Were Gabriel's pictures simply pictures? Should we allow Tommy to snuggle with the same scarf he had just used to try to strangle himself? Was there no way to help Jasmine calm down other than locked leather restraints? Can we really let the boy suffering from disabling OCD walk out of the APS because he did not meet commitment criteria? The answer: it depends—sometimes pictures are harmless expressions of developmentally appropriate emotions, sometimes they are expressions of inappropriate or even malicious intent. As caregivers who want to make a difference, we try to learn as much as possible about the child in front of us, muster the limited resources available in the system, make safety our priority, and hope for the best.

GLOSSARY

51A: the report of abuse or neglect of a minor made to the Department of Children and Families (DCF). It is called a 51A because Section 51A of Massachusetts General Law Chapter 119 requires certain professionals, called "mandated reporters," to report reasonable concerns of abuse or neglect to DCF. Completing this report is called "filing a 51A," or more simply "filing."

Asperger's disorder: a disorder on the mild end of the autism spectrum characterized by social difficulties, rigid behavior, and intense interest in a particular subject.

Attending: a doctor on the hospital staff who has completed residency and is board-eligible or certified to practice his or her specialty independently.

Bay: also known as a holding room, a room within the APS containing only a stretcher with a door that can be locked if necessary.

Bullycide: suicide by someone who is the victim of bullying.

Child in Need of Services (CHINS): a legal proceeding in which a parent or a school files a petition asking the juvenile court to help a child or an adolescent with problematic behavior. The behavior needs to fall into one of four categories: frequent running away, refusal to obey the rules of the parents, regularly failing to attend school, or persistent violation of school rules. When the CHINS petition is filed with the court, the child is assigned a probation officer, who determines the rules and services that will be put into place by the court with the goal of changing the child's behavior.

Child psychiatry resident: also known as a child psychiatry fellow, a doctor who has completed an adult psychiatry residency and is participating in a fellowship program for advanced training in child psychiatry.

Children's Behavioral Health Initiative (CBHI): an interagency initiative in Massachusetts to expand community-based mental health services for children and families with the goal of maintaining children in the community and avoiding hospitalizations.

Cognitive behavioral therapy (CBT): a type of psychotherapy that uses a highly structured, goal-oriented, systematic approach to treat a variety of psychiatric disorders. It is a time-limited therapy that focuses on the link between thoughts, feelings, and behaviors.

Commit: hospitalizing a patient in a psychiatric unit against his or her will (see also Section 12).

Computer biopsy: also known as a chart biopsy, a review of all notes and testing results in a patient's electronic medical record.

CRAFFT screen: a six-item questionnaire used to screen for alcohol and drug use in adolescents between 12 and 18 years old.

Delirium: a syndrome characterized by acute onset of attention deficits, disorientation, and confusion, as well as fluctuating level of consciousness.

Department of Children and Families (DCF): The Department of Children and Families, formerly known as the Department of Social Services (DSS), is the state agency charged with protecting children from abuse and neglect in the Commonwealth of Massachusetts.

Department of Youth Services (DYS): the juvenile justice agency of the Commonwealth of Massachusetts. This agency oversees all youth in the correctional system for the state.

Developmental pediatrician: a pediatrician who specializes in the diagnosis and treatment of children with developmental delays and disabilities.

ED: Emergency Department.

Electroencepahologram (EEG): the recording of the brain's electrical activity by placing multiple electrodes on the scalp. An EEG can be used to diagnose epilepsy, among other neurologic illnesses.

Emergency Medical Treatment and Active Labor Act (EMTALA): requires emergency medical treatment for all patients, regardless of their citizenships legal status, or ability to pay; also mandates that patients may only be transferred or discharged after they have been stabilized and have consented, or if they are going to a facility better able to manage their particular needs.

Fellow: a doctor who has completed residency and is participating in a fellowship program for advanced training in a particular subspecialty, such as child psychiatry.

Individualized Education Program (IEP): special instruction and support services designed to allow children with a disability (physical, emotional, intellectual) to access the general school curriculum. Commonly known as special education, the goal is to support children so they may achieve up to their academic potential. Each child has a unique IEP based on his or her individual needs.

Inpatient unit: also called simply inpatient, a locked psychiatric unit capable of managing acute crisis, with an average stay lasting 1–2 weeks.

Intermittent explosive disorder: a disorder characterized by explosions of anger that are disproportionate to the situation.

Intramuscular (IM): a route of administering medication directly into the muscle by injection.

Junior resident: (see resident) a resident in his or her second year of training.

Neuropsychological testing: extensive testing done by a skilled examiner to ascertain a patient's IQ, learning strengths and weakness, psychological tendencies and conflicts, among other measures.

OCD: obsessive compulsive disorder.

Outpatient: any type of treatment a patient receives outside of a psychiatric ward.

Paradoxical response: when a patient has the opposite response to a medication than what is typical. Most frequently, this refers to children who become activated from medications that are typically sedating.

Patient advocacy: the office that assists patients in voicing and managing complaints and concerns about their care at the hospital.

Pediatric autoimmune neuropsychiatric disorder associated with streptococcal infections (PANDAS): an illness similar to OCD in which antibodies triggered by a streptococcal infection attack the parts of the brain that are thought to control obsessions, compulsions, and tics.

Pink paper: colloquial term for the Section 12 form. It is called a "pink paper" because the Section 12 is typically printed on bright pink paper.

PO: the Latin *per os* means "by mouth," referring to medications given orally.

Psychology intern: a clinician who has completed graduate school in psychology and is in the process of completing his or her dissertation. On completion of the dissertation and the requisite clinical hours, the clinician will become a psychologist.

Repeat offender: a colloquialism for any patient with multiple presentations to the ED.

Resident: a doctor who has completed medical school and is enrolled in a residency program to learn a specialty, for example, psychiatry.

Residential treatment program: also known as resi, a residential (meaning the patients stay overnight) treatment program with a length of stay measured in months, not days or weeks. These programs are not locked, and all patients are voluntary.

Patients are typically more stable than those on inpatient units, and most of these admissions are not covered by insurance.

Restraint: any manual method or mechanical device that immobilizes or reduces the ability of a patient to move freely.

Seclusion: involuntary confinement of a patient alone in a room that he or she is physically prevented from leaving.

Section 12: a Section 12a is an order signed by a physician to have a mentally ill patient transported, held, and evaluated in an Emergency Department due to concern that the individual is at substantial risk of harming him or herself, harming someone else, or is unable to care for him or herself. The order is based on Section 12 of Massachusetts General Law Chapter 123. After the evaluation, if the patient is still deemed to be at substantial risk, he or she can be admitted involuntarily to a psychiatric unit for up to 72 hours under a Section 12b signed by a physician at the designated facility.

Senior resident: (see resident) a resident in his or her third or fourth year of training.

Suicidal ideation (SI): having thoughts of committing suicide.

Three day: also known as three-day notice, a signed notice from a patient currently admitted to an inpatient unit that he or she wishes to be discharged. The doctor then has up to three business days to decide if it is safe to release the patient or to go to court to obtain a commitment order.

Tox screen: a test of the serum or urine to determine what, if any, drugs the patient has ingested recently.

Triage: the initial screening area of the emergency department where a triage nurse evaluates all new patients. The nurse takes a brief history and checks the patient's vital signs. Based on the condition of the patient, the triage nurse will then send the patient to the appropriate area of the ED.

Urine tox: see tox screen.

INDEX

About the Authors

LAURA M. PRAGER, MD, is an assistant professor of psychiatry (child psychiatry) at Harvard Medical School and the director of the Child Psychiatry Emergency Service at Massachusetts General Hospital. She is an assistant editor for the *Journal of the American Academy of Child and Adolescent Psychiatry* and a reviewer for the journals *Pediatrics, Critical Care Medicine, Journal of Developmental and Behavioral Pediatrics,* and *Psychosomatics.* Dr. Prager has authored and coauthored articles in *Harvard Review of Psychiatry, Psychiatric Times, Journal of the American Academy of Child and Adolescent Psychiatry, JAMA,* and others, as well as chapters in books published by Mosby, Elsevier, and the American Academy of Pediatrics. Dr. Prager has won numerous awards for teaching from the Department of Child Psychiatry at Massachusetts General Hospital.

ABIGAIL L. DONOVAN, MD, is an assistant psychiatrist at Massachusetts General Hospital and a clinical instructor of psychiatry at Harvard Medical School. She is the associate director of the Acute Psychiatry Service at Massachusetts General Hospital. She is also a core member of the teaching faculty for both the adult and child and adolescent psychiatry residencies at Massachusetts General Hospital. Dr. Donovan has authored and coauthored articles in *Proceedings of the National Academy of Sciences, Pediatrics,* and the *Journal of Clinical Psychiatry,* as well as numerous book chapters. She is a former member of the Board of Trustees of the American Psychiatric Association. Dr. Donovan has been nominated for a Brian A. McGovern award for clinical excellence.

About the Series Editor

JULIE SILVER, MD, is assistant professor, Harvard Medical School, Department of Physical Medicine and Rehabilitation, and is on the medical staff at Brigham & Women's, Massachusetts General and Spaulding Rehabilitation Hospitals in Boston, Massachusetts. Dr. Silver has authored, edited, or coedited dozens of books, including medical textbooks and consumer health guides. She is also the chief editor of books at Harvard Health Publications. Dr. Silver has won many awards, including the American Medical Writers Association Solimene Award for Excellence in Medical Writing and the prestigious Lane Adams Quality of Life Award from the American Cancer Society. Silver teaches health care providers how to write and publish, and she is the director of an annual course offered by the Harvard Medical School Department of Continuing Education titled Publishing Books, Memoirs and Other Creative Non-Fiction. For more about her work, visit www.JulieSilverMD.com.